Timeless SKIN

Splash Publishing

healthy

skin

for a

lifetime

Carolyn ASH

Copyright © 2000 by Carolyn Ash

Published by Splash Publishing
Post Office Box 720177
Dallas, Texas 75372

Illustrations by Narda Lebo
Cover photography by Tom Hussey

Library of Congress Cataloging-in-Publication Data
Ash, Carolyn
   Timeless skin: healthy skin for a lifetime/Carolyn Ash.
      p.   cm.
   Includes index & illustrations
   ISBN 0-9670240-0-5
   1. Skin care   2. Beauty   3. Health   I. Title
Library of Congress Catalog Number: 99-93759

Printed in the United States of America

10% of the net proceeds from this First Edition will be donated to the American Cancer Society. Thank you for your purchase.

C O N T E N T S

A C K N O W L E D G M E N T S

I am indebted to: Mary Stilwell, Carol Considine, Steve Gibbs, Narda Lebo, Julie Flandorfer, Mel Ann Coley, Tom Hussey, Bill Robinson, Melissa Gioldasis

Special thanks to: My family, my family of clients, Lisa Loeb, Merry Vose, Barbara Ferguson, Yvonne O'Brien, Gigi Sussman, Mary Bland, Sharon Kraus, Deborah Keller, Teel Lunsford, Sharon Thompson, Katharine Bernard, Katherine Collop, Johnson & Johnson, Bob Hoffman, Velma J. Keith & Monteen Gordon, the American Cancer Society, Publishers Press

I am dedicating *Timeless Skin* to my clients—those I have seen through the years and those of you I have yet to meet. Few books have been written by those of us working with skin on a day-to-day basis, so I wanted to write about my experience with skin as a licensed aesthetician (someone who gives facials) and to give practical information to help keep your skin healthy— inside and out. I have tried to tell you everything I share with my clients in an easy-to-follow and instructional format. I realize some of this information will contradict what you have always heard to be true, and that's OK. I have developed my own particular style and philosophy of caring for skin that I believe you will find informative and indeed beneficial.

Everyone who comes to see me has individual needs, yet there are common denominators in treating all skin conditions. I believe you will be able to glean pieces of information and put together a skin care program that works for you. Read through the whole book, and then keep it handy as a reference guide, looking things up as needed.

I did not necessarily separate information for different races, genders, or even ages since I treat all individuals as unique, no matter who they are. Also, there are a few instances where I refer to an individual as "she" or "her." This is not to exclude any men who are reading this book. These words were simply used to avoid the use of he/she and him/her.

I hope that after reading *Timeless Skin*, you will start to question the sometimes overwhelming abundance of information on skin care so that you can discern truth from fiction. My goal is to break down the seemingly impenetrable structure that makes up our Fountain of Youth mythology, presenting instead information that leads you down a path to reality. The truth usually makes good sense, and it is my hope that this book gives you the freedom to pay less attention to all the hype and to help your skin be its best—for a lifetime.

I hope you enjoy reading *Timeless Skin* as much as I enjoyed writing it.

Be Well,

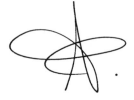

"Nature gives you the face you have at twenty; it is up to you to merit the face you have at fifty."

—Coco Chanel

The Basics

Skin care doesn't have to be complicated. It also doesn't require a lot of time. The best results will be found by being consistent. Your basic daily routine consists of three steps. Step 1: Cleansing, Step 2: Toning, and Step 3: Moisturizing. Eye cream is important, and I consider it part of the moisturizing step. You can get by just doing The Basics 1-2-3 every day in the morning and evening, but there are a few extras I highly recommend, which are discussed in Chapter 2.

Before we get into the basics about caring for your skin, I want to address a few important points you may not be aware of. First, I hear a lot of people say, "My skin can't breathe," or after removing a heavy cream or foundation, "Now my skin *can* breathe." Well, the truth is your skin doesn't breathe. Not externally, anyway. Your skin is nourished from the oxygen and nutrients carried in the blood. By diffusing through the blood vessels or capillary walls, oxygen enters the cells while toxins are expelled into the bloodstream. But no measurable amount of oxygen is absorbed from the outside air. However, your skin does eliminate toxins, sweat, and oil and absorbs moisture from the air. When you put on a heavy cream or foundation your skin is less able to function properly, and you might mistakenly say it "can't breathe." These occlusive coverings can inhibit elimination and absorption, but not the actual oxygen nourishing your skin.

Next, you always want to use tepid water on your face—never hot or cold. Tepid means lukewarm, neutral, or moderate in terms of temperature. The vascular system for your face is made up of tiny vessels (capillaries), which by nature are very weak. I once heard a doctor say, "Capillaries are akin to wet toilet paper." Now *that's* weak! Extremes in temperature are often too much for the capillaries to tolerate, causing couperose (broken capillaries), redness, and sensitivity. When you're in the shower, turn away from the water. Let it drip down your face, as opposed to sticking your face in the hot shower spray. Or you can cup your hands and splash-rinse, giving the hot water a chance to cool off before it hits your face. Either way, keep your face out of the direct spray of hot water. Cold water is equally damaging to the delicate capillaries.

In addition to avoiding temperature extremes, it's a good idea to keep shampoo and other hair products off your face. To rinse products out of your hair, stand with your face away from the shower and tilt your head back with your hands acting as a barrier along your hairline.

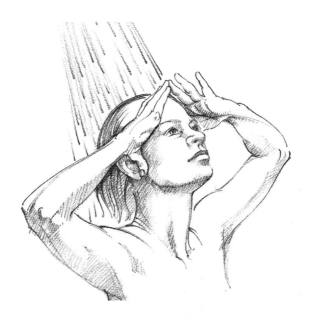

With your hands acting as a barrier, hot water and hair products are kept off your face in the shower.

Rinsing your hair this way will ensure these products don't get on your facial skin. It's not the end of the world, but the ingredients in hair products could potentially cause irritation, so why risk it?

Also, always use your skin care products on your neck as well as your face. Although the tissue on your neck is different (fewer oil glands, thinner skin), it still responds to care and will show signs of neglect. So include your neck in everything you do. (See Chapter 12/The Forgotten Places.)

Finally, *hypoallergenic, dermatologist-tested,* and *allergy-free* are all unregulated terms. In some cases, these terms just mean a team of dermatologists got together and determined for themselves what did and did not cause skin to break out or become sensitive to a particular product. There are no guidelines set by the Food & Drug Administration (FDA) governing which products can say they are hypoallergenic, etc. Products with these descriptions are simply less likely to produce a reaction. You still may find yourself sensitive to a product, allergy-free or not. Ultimately, you'll have to try the product before you'll know if it will work for you. A product claiming to be *non-comedogenic* won't (or shouldn't) clog your pores.

Now I want to walk you through The Basics one step at a time. This routine should only take one or two minutes to complete unless you enjoy spending more time caring for your skin. Three basic steps, that's all it is.

Step 1: Cleansing

What is a cleanser? A cleanser is a product that helps to remove oil and debris from the surface of your skin. Cleansers usually contain wetting agents called surfactants. These agents enable the oil and water from your skin to mix together to be washed away as you rinse the product off. Cleansing milks are primarily water with an oil or fat included in the ingredients, which renders them oil-in-water emulsions. Cold creams, with their primary ingredient usually a form of mineral oil or a petroleum derivative, are termed water-in-oil emulsions. Soaps come in bars and liquids and contain detergents and foaming agents—ingredients that get your skin squeaky clean.

Cleansers are *not* moisturizers. Some cleansing products claim to leave your skin feeling "soft and moisturized." Softening the skin is fine, but your moisturizing cream is what remains on the surface to hydrate your skin. A cleanser is applied and removed. It should not leave any type of film on the skin to moisturize. This remaining film could potentially clog the pores causing congestion problems in the future. Cleansers cleanse; they do not (or should not) remain on the skin.

Why cleanse? Cleansing is the most important step in your daily program. If you don't get your skin clean, everything else you do will be less effective. It's like putting wax on your car without thoroughly washing it first. The skin needs to remain clean to maintain the integrity of the pores, and using a cleanser is the best way to achieve this. If you don't cleanse, you're doing your skin a huge disservice. You could be setting up an environment for clogged and therefore enlarged pores as well as amassing a thick, dead skin buildup that can also contribute to congestion. Just imagine not brushing your teeth for a few days, and you'll see what I mean.

What to use. Your skin is naturally acidic on the pH scale. *pH* refers to how acid or alkaline a substance is. The scale ranges from 0 to 14, with 7 being neutral. Your skin has a pH of 5 or 6; soaps usually come in around 10. In order to maintain the natural acidic state of your skin, you always want to use acidic or non-alkaline products. If you are unsure about the pH of your cleanser (or any product), you can purchase nitrazine papers at your local pharmacy.

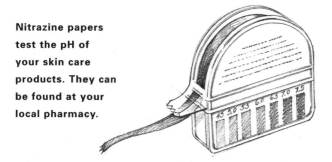

Nitrazine papers test the pH of your skin care products. They can be found at your local pharmacy.

These yellowish test papers come in a roll about 1/4" wide. (Be aware, they can be expensive. I recently paid $20 for one roll, which was nearly double what I paid five years ago. See Quick Tips at the end of this chapter.) Dip a small piece into any jar or bottle, or pour a bit of any substance onto the paper. You'll find out immediately if the product is alkaline or acid. This is very important to know. You never want to use alkaline products on your face. If your research finds a product you're using is alkaline, I would toss it. Don't bother trying to make it work for your skin. It won't. Although the department stores abhor people testing their products, take your nitrazine papers whenever you plan to purchase products.

You want to use a cleanser that gently removes surface oil and debris off your face; you don't ever want to "strip" the skin. Water-soluble cleansers are best. *Water-soluble* means it dissolves in water. Most milk cleansers and washes are water-soluble, but cold creams are not. Cold creams tend to leave a film on the skin because the oils are not broken down by merely rinsing with water. In addition, cold creams are usually tissued off, which guarantees a coating of oil will be left on the skin. For people with drier skin types, this film usually won't cause problems. But for those of you with normal to oily or problem skin, any product left on the surface could cause trouble. I would advise you to avoid thick cold creams, and no matter what type of cleanser you are using, always rinse your face with water (splash-rinse).

By the way, water-soluble cleansers generally do not lather. They don't contain the harsh and drying ingredients of bar soap, so they may not foam up. If they're acidic, which is what you're looking for, they also won't strip the skin. If you're a soap user and not used to this non-lathering type of cleanser, give it time. You may have to go through an adjustment period before you feel these kinder, gentler, water-soluble cleansers are working, but they are.

I'm not a fan of soap as a general rule. The ingredients used to make it a hard bar are harsh and better kept off your face. You may feel soap gets your skin squeaky clean—and you're right. But soap gets it *too* clean. So in reality, you've just stripped all the oil and all the water off the surface of your skin. This will give you a taut feeling (which you may associate with clean), but your skin is now stripped! You don't have to strip everything off in order to get a good, general cleanse. And when your skin is stripped, it is left vulnerable until the proper pH is restored. It's as though you're moving out of your house or apartment, and you not only take all your belongings and furniture, but you also pull up the carpet, take the wallpaper down, and peel the paint from the walls. Soap has a similar effect on your skin.

If you must use soap, try a brand called Aveeno®. Although this is a non-alkaline soap, it still may leave your skin feeling dried out. I recommend Aveeno to clients who have to use soap, teenagers who don't have the resources to purchase more expensive cleansers, or clients with problem skin who sometimes feel milk cleansers are not getting their skin clean. I still prefer cleansing milks, but if you have to use soap, try Aveeno. It also comes in a liquid "oil control formula." Cetaphil® is another brand that makes a liquid "gentle skin cleanser." Both of these liquid cleansers are non-alkaline (and inexpensive) and don't seem to dry out the skin the way bar soaps do.

How to cleanse. Once you know your cleanser is OK to use, put a reasonable amount in the palm of your hand. If you have a milk cleanser, use about the size of a quarter to a half-dollar. With foaming cleansers, you'll only need half as much. Put your palms together so the cleanser spreads evenly on both hands and gently go over your entire face and neck. You are not rubbing hard, your hands are merely gliding over your skin. Many skin care regimens get picky about exactly how to do each step, like "splash 15 times with water captured in your basin" or "only use counterclockwise circles when applying products." Instead of focusing on which way your hands are moving across your face, my main concern is getting you in the habit of using your cleanser. As long as you don't pull the skin, use circular motion or whatever feels most effective. Don't forget to get the cleanser in that ridge between your earlobe and cheek as well as behind your ears. Dirt and debris tend to collect in these odd places, and you want to clean them daily, too.

After you have massaged the cleanser onto your skin (this should only take 10 or 15 seconds), remove it by splash-rinsing with tepid water. Pat your skin dry with a towel (again, no rubbing), and you're clean and ready for Step 2: Toning.

You may be wondering if you should add water to your cleanser. The effectiveness of the cleanser is not contingent on how wet or dry your skin is. In this instance, let your personal preference be your guide. Some people like to put cleanser on a wet face, either in the shower or at the sink. You may prefer to apply it to your dry skin. Personally, I choose to add a little water to my cleanser, which allows it to glide across my face.

A word about washcloths: I'm not a big fan. They harbor bacteria and can put extra drag on the skin without your ever noticing. Although the rough terry cloth will exfoliate some dead cells off the surface of your skin, I recommend actively exfoliating with a product instead of relying on a washcloth to do this work. If you're rubbing your skin hard enough with a washcloth to get any significant exfoliation, you are rubbing your face too hard. When you use your hands to cleanse and wash away products, you can tell by touch if everything is off your skin. You also get a feel for your skin on a twice-daily basis. You can tell if there are any blemishes or unusual bumps that you wouldn't be able to feel through a thick piece of cloth. If you choose to use washcloths, just don't rub too hard and make sure to use a clean one every time.

When to cleanse. You should cleanse both morning and evening. The need to cleanse in the evening may seem a bit obvious if you've been wearing makeup all day. But even if you don't wear makeup, you still have a buildup of debris, sweat, and oil as well as pollution from the environment that needs to be removed. Even though your body goes into a more regenerative (less active) mode overnight, you still want to wash your face in the morning. This way you'll have a fresh, clean start to your day. You clean your teeth in the morning even though you brushed them the night before, and you should clean your skin too.

A big mistake makeup wearers make is to not clean their skin thoroughly. It's not enough to just remove the day's makeup, you must also clean the skin underneath. If you wear makeup, you'll want to cleanse twice at night. Once to get the makeup off, and the second time to get your skin clean. And don't get me started on those of you who don't wash your makeup off at night. I didn't write much about this subject assuming you already know it's bad to sleep with makeup on.

Step 2: Toning

What is a toner? Toner (also called freshener, astringent, clarifying lotion, etc.) is a water-based liquid designed to superficially hydrate and lower the pH of the skin. Almost all product lines have toners. Read further to find out why you want to use toner, how to use one, and what to watch out for.

Why use a toner? Toners are an important yet misunderstood step in your daily program. You may have heard they are the second step in cleansing: "Wipe your face with a cotton ball soaked in toner and look at all the dirt it picks up." What that really means is you didn't get your skin clean, so it's back to Step 1: Cleansing for you. Cleansers cleanse, toners tone or prepare the skin. Toners are *not* cleansers. Technically, toners reacidify the epidermis and prepare the skin for moisturizer. To *reacidify* means to replace the skin's naturally low (acidic) pH, which is disrupted somewhat even with gentle cleansers. *Epidermis* is just another word for your outer, dead skin, the skin you can touch. So toners help replace the natural acidic state of your skin. Toners are primarily water, so they also superficially hydrate the outer skin. After cleansing and toning, you are ready for Step 3: Moisturizing, discussed a bit later.

Some of you may be using toners thinking you are tightening or even shrinking your pores. Unfortunately, this is not the case. It is physiologically impossible to shrink the pores. (See Chapter 16/Myth: Pores shrink.) Toners that have alcohol or other drying agents in them cause your skin to swell slightly, giving you the feeling of tightening. But actually these drying agents (especially alcohol) will *strip* the skin and eventually cause dehydration—making your skin feel dry. Toners prepare the skin for moisturizing, they do not alter the structure of the skin.

What to use. First of all, you don't ever want to use a toner with SD, Ethyl, or Isopropyl Alcohol. SD stands for *specially denatured;* denatured renders it undrinkable. (A bittering agent is added to the alcohol so people won't accidentally drink it.) Ethyl and Isopropyl Alcohol (also known as Rubbing Alcohol) are very drying and not good ingredients for promoting healthy skin. Cetyl alcohol, on the other hand, is a waxy, emollient ingredient found in many cosmetic preparations and is not harmful to the skin. Not all alcohols are bad, just the ones listed above.

Years ago many toners contained alcohol, but it's not as prevalent an ingredient today. It was thought back then that drying the skin out with alcohol would help dry up oily skin. On the surface, that sounds good. You're producing a lot of oil, so surely the answer is to get rid of that oily buildup. Unfortunately, running a cotton ball with an alcohol-based toner over your face is just removing the symptom—the excess oil. And it will undoubtedly cause another problem—dehydration. You need to affect the cause of the problem (overactive oil glands) before you can stop producing the symptom (oily skin). In other words, alcohol or any drying agent is simply drying up the oil, not stopping the oil glands from overproducing.

The cause of a skin condition is usually varied and complex, so treating the symptom seems the easier road to take. But in the end, only treating the symptom can create more problems. And so it is with alcohol. Like other alkaline products, alcohol strips every particle of oil and water off the surface of your skin, leaving it bare and imbalanced. Your oil glands will tend to pump out more oil to overcompensate for the loss, which causes the potential for even oilier skin than you started with. And because you're removing all the oil and water off the surface, your skin will most likely become dehydrated too. This is all very bad news. Supple, hydrated, well-nourished skin is what you're after. Using toners with alcohol in them will give you the opposite effect. Just say no to alcohol!

When looking for a toner, I would seek out an ingredient list that is short and without a lot of long, chemical-sounding names. The shorter the ingredient list, the better. Why? Because a long ingredient list equals a more complex substance; therefore, the chances are greater for irritation or intolerances. As with the foods you eat, simple is best. Complex dishes, sauces, and soups made with lots of different ingredients can cause indigestion. There are just too many components for the digestive system to handle. Your skin is really no different. It likes simple, moderate, and gentle products used on it. Water should be (and usually is) the first ingredient in your alcohol-free toner.

Finally, find a toner with an aroma that is appealing to you. Toner remains on the skin, so how it smells will affect your desire to use it or not. Be careful it is not ladened with synthetic fragrance. As discussed in Chapter 15, fragrance can cause problems for your skin. Essential oils (lavender, rosemary, cypress, to name a few) make good ingredients for a toner. They are naturally acidic as well as wonderfully (naturally) aromatic. (See Chapter 8/Essential Oils.)

How to use toner. Most likely you have always put toner on a cotton pad and gone over your face with it. Or you may have been splashing it on like an aftershave. I recommend spraying toner on your face as the optimum way of applying it. This method is quick, economical, and the most effective way to apply toner evenly onto

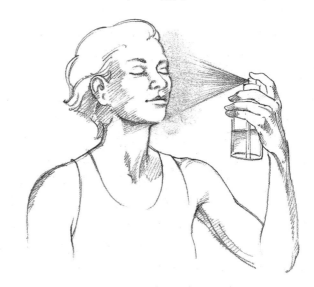

Put your toner in a spray bottle for a quick and effective application. Empty spray bottles can easily be found at the grocery store.

your face. It feels refreshing as well, and you don't need to keep cotton around. Men certainly don't want to mess with cotton, having to inevitably spend time picking tiny strings of it out of their beards. Empty spray bottles are easy to find at any beauty supply or grocery store.

When to tone. Always use a toner after cleansing. Because you have slightly disrupted the pH of your skin while cleansing, you want to reacidify the surface. Using toner after cleansing sets up the right environment for your skin to be balanced and then prepared for hydration (moisturizing). Your toner should be gentle enough that you can spray it throughout the day. Whenever I go into my bathroom, I grab my toner and enjoy a refreshing spray mist. It's a wonderful little treat for my face. In general, however, after you have thoroughly washed your face and neck (morning and evening) and patted your skin dry with a towel, use your toner. On to your third and final step, moisturizing.

Step 3: Moisturizing

What is a moisturizer? A moisturizer (also called a hydrating cream or lotion) is an emollient oil-in-water mixture, usually a cream (sometimes a gel), that is spread over the skin to help lock in moisture. Moisturizers generally contain a humectant (an ingredient that draws moisture to itself) to further hydrate the skin. Moisturizers, whether for the face or specifically for the eye area, do not erase or in any measurable way reduce lines and wrinkles. They may lessen the *appearance* of lines, but that is all they are equipped to do.

Why use a moisturizer? Moisturizers add a layer of protection between your skin and the outside environment. They help to plump up dead skin cells, which gives the appearance of reducing fine, superficial lines (wrinkles). They also make your skin feel smooth and well hydrated. If you have true-dry skin (skin that doesn't emit enough oil, explained further in Chapter 4), you already know a moisturizer's importance. Without one, your skin would feel like a flaking, cracking desert. People with dry skin need to make up for the lack of oil in their skin and moisturizers serve that purpose.

Those of you with oily skin may have trouble understanding why you should use a moisturizer—or if you need to use one at all. Using a poor-quality moisturizer on problem or oily skin can indeed cause problems. But this doesn't mean all moisturizers are bad for oilier skin types. My belief is that practically everyone needs a moisturizer. Even people with acne need to hydrate their skin. In fact, those of you with problem skin usually have very dehydrated and depleted skin as well as blemishes. The constant use of harsh and drying products that attempt to dry out the oil can really do a number on the skin.

There definitely is a controversy surrounding the use of moisturizers on oily skin. If your skin seems excessively oily and you don't feel you need a moisturizer, ask yourself these questions:

(1) Do I use soap or a harsh cleanser that may be stripping my skin? (2) Do I use a toner with alcohol in it? (3) Do I use blemish pads that help to "dry up" excess oil? If the answer is "yes" to any of these questions, your skin might be pumping out more oil than it normally would due to all those drying agents. Test your products with nitrazine papers to make sure they are acidic. If they aren't, consider throwing them out and find others that are non-alkaline. After using these gentler products, see if you have less trouble with oiliness. Then find a light-textured moisturizer to use day and night to complete your 1-2-3 program.

If your products are acidic and are not drying out your skin, yet you still produce a lot of oil, you may not need a moisturizer. Your diet could be a factor, you may be predisposed genetically to oily skin, or perhaps your hormones are imbalanced. This would be a good time to seek out a professional facial (see Chapter 3) and hear what a licensed specialist has to say. If you truly feel you don't need to use a moisturizer, although I hesitate to say this, then don't use one.

I hesitate because without a moisturizing cream, you leave your skin's surface vulnerable to the environment. Without the protection of a cream or gel, dirt and debris can find their way deeper into your pores. And without adequate moisture on the surface, your oil glands may feel the need to pump out more oil than necessary to compensate for the dryness. Finally, high-quality products contain ingredients to combat the oiliness and can actually help tackle the problem. Clients with very oily skin often cringe when I suggest they use a moisturizer. I can usually convince them to at least try one for a few days after explaining my position. Hydrating gels are an alternative to creams, giving you protection without adding oil.

What to use. Using a cream that is made for your particular skin type is of great importance. If you use an inappropriate product, you can really cause problems. Moisturizers (and toners) stay on your skin day and night, whereas cleansers go on briefly and come right off.

Acidic or non-alkaline moisturizers are what you want to use because they will not disrupt the natural balance of your skin. Bacteria do not thrive in an acid environment, so using a moisturizer that is acidic on the pH scale can go a long way in keeping bacteria at bay. Pure essential oils (see Chapter 8/Essential Oils) are acidic by nature, so they make good ingredients in skin care products. Test your moisturizer with nitrazine papers to be sure it's OK to use. Be aware that just because the test results show your cream is acidic, there is no guarantee it will be effective in clearing up problem skin. But it's a good start.

What about the term *oil-free*? Unfortunately, this is one of those instances where being a chemist would be of great help. Many oil-free products contain no oil, but employ filler and emollient ingredients that can clog your pores just like an oil. It's similar to fat-free foods that don't have a high fat content, but are loaded with carbohydrates that are stored in your body as fat. Tricky, isn't it?

If you have oily skin, you should avoid petroleum products. Petroleum-based ingredients (mineral oil, petroleum jelly, paraffin) can be very clogging. They have a large molecular structure and just sit on the surface inhibiting proper skin function (elimination and absorption) and can leave a greasy film. If you have true-dry skin, you won't have as many problems using these poor-quality ingredients as a person with problem skin will.

Oils aren't altogether bad. And although you don't want to use heavy creams on oily skin, all oils are not to be avoided. Vegetal oils have a small molecular structure and are easily absorbed by your outer skin. These oils tend to be lighter in texture, making the moisturizer less oily to the touch. Vegetal oils have nutrients in them, whereas petroleum products are basically nutrient-deficient.

If you consistently experience burning or itching soon after applying your moisturizing cream (or *any* product), I suggest immediately removing it and tossing it in the garbage. Better yet, return it for a full refund. These types of reactions are your skin telling you it has an intolerance to something contained in the product. Burning and itching are not normal responses and should be regarded as warning signs. Narrowing down ingredients you're allergic or intolerant to can help you further down the road when shopping for products. Finally, not all moisturizers are good for your skin, no matter how much money you spend on them.

Day vs. night. Many people are confused over the use of day and night creams. What is the difference? Do you really need to use two different products on your skin? The answer is both yes and no. Function and variety are the two main reasons for using a different moisturizer on your face during the day and at night.

Day creams add a blanket of protection to your skin from the outside environment. This not only includes guarding against sunlight (if your day cream has a built-in sunscreen) but also dirt and debris in the air. A moisturizer will add a layer of protection between your skin and any makeup you may be wearing. These creams also supply oil and nutrients to the skin to help keep it soft, supple, and moisturized.

Night creams are usually more treatment oriented than their day cream counterparts. Nighttime is when your body (and your skin) goes into a less active, more regenerative and repairing mode. Night creams are generally made to address specific needs that your protective day creams may not and are generally not meant to be worn under makeup.

Another reason to use two different creams is variety. Your skin can benefit from the variety of ingredients in two creams, instead of constantly using just one. Also there is the added benefit of diversity of aromas and textures. Using the same cream day and night limits you on these levels as well. This may not be important to you, but many people like to have a variety of experiences when it comes to the way their creams smell and feel.

I recommend using a different cream for day and for night. You will benefit from a variety of ingredients and actions, as well as different aromas and textures. But if using one cream both day and night works best for you (many of my clients fall into this category), it is surely not harmful to use one cream. As long as the moisturizer you are using is appropriate for your skin type, this simpler approach is perfectly all right.

How to moisturize. When applying moisturizer, you may put dots of cream on different parts of your face and then smooth them in. I propose an alternate way to apply your moisturizer. Although it's a small change, it can make a big difference. Put a peanut-sized dollop in the palm of one hand, then rub your hands together to emulsify and warm the cream. Smooth the cream over your entire face and neck using both your hands (palms), not just the tips of your fingers. Applying the moisturizer this way increases your chances of getting the cream on all parts of your face evenly. This is important. The connect-the-dot method can cause an uneven application; some areas will have a concentration of moisturizer while others will hardly have any.

If your nose tends to get oily during the day, bypass it when applying the cream. Just lightly go over the nose area as you finish smoothing the cream over your face and neck. This should help to keep the oily nose syndrome to a minimum. Also, if you have to pat off excess product from your face, you've used too much. Try using less cream to start with, then while your face is still wet from the toner, apply your moisturizer. This will help you achieve a thinner application.

When to moisturize. You always want to apply a moisturizer after cleansing and toning (Steps 1 & 2). You also want to use it both in the morning and at night. Usually, moisturizer is the last product you put on your skin. If you are wearing foundation, it will go on top of your day cream. The next section on eye cream is a continuation of Step 3, but it specifically addresses caring for the under-eye area.

Eye Cream

What is eye cream? The skin around the eyes and on the eyelids is the thinnest skin on your body. Eye creams provide a lipid or emollient substance to keep this delicate tissue soft. So eye cream is essentially a moisturizer formulated specifically for the skin around your eyes. Eye creams do not erase wrinkles or prevent them from coming. They can soften the look of the lines and help to decrease the *appearance* of wrinkles, but not the wrinkles themselves. Eye cream is important, but not magical.

Why use eye cream? You have no functioning oil glands directly under your eyes, so you want to keep that skin moisturized at all times. Why? So that when you express and the lines crease around your eyes, they are creasing on soft tissue. Lines are formed after years of facial expressions and sun exposure that cause a breakdown of collagen (the supporting structure of the skin), which then creates a wrinkle. A topical cream is merely keeping the tissue soft and, therefore, the lines less noticeable—less hard looking. Creams cannot repair damage induced by sun exposure, nor can a cream stop the natural aging process. At best, with eye creams specifically, they can help to soften the blow caused by facial expressions.

As consumers, we have been lulled into believing a mere man-made cream can overturn what nature, genetics, and sun exposure have caused. Don't be fooled. Being clear about what is and what is not possible will save you a lot of time and money. However, using eye creams is vitally important in keeping the tissue around the eye area soft and supple, reducing the look of the lines.

What to use. Eye creams are very important, but don't get ripped off buying an expensive one. Manufacturers know how important they are (and how concerned you are about wrinkles), so they tend to gouge you, charging exorbitant prices for a tiny tube or jar of eye cream. Although these creams are formulated specifically for the delicate tissue around the eyes, it is unnecessary to pay $50, $70, or even $90 for an eye cream.

There are eye creams on the market designed to reduce puffiness and even dark circles. These may help in some cases, but if you have chronic problems around the eyes, no cream is going to eradicate them. If you have inherited dark circles, you can buy as many creams as you want to, but nothing is really going to make the darkness go away. If edema (puffiness) is your problem and if this is inherited, nothing short of surgery will do much in the way of getting rid of the puffiness. I am not advocating surgery, I just don't want you to get your hopes up when looking for miracles in a simple jar of cream. If your under-eye problems are minor ones, using these types of special eye creams may indeed help.

If you are sensitive around the eye area (most people are), you obviously want to find a cream that causes no sensation (irritation, stinging, burning). Fragrance is *out* as far as an ingredient in your eye cream. It can irritate even nonsensitive skin. Sometimes product sensitivities can cause puffiness, so be careful.

You can't always sample eye creams. Many companies don't make samples available, probably because eye creams come in such small containers as it is. Check the ingredient list and make sure there is no fragrance. Then, if you can, test the eye cream right then and there at the cosmetic counter or facial salon. If you are going to have a reaction, it usually doesn't take long. If the cream feels good and is reasonably priced, try it out.

Gels vs. creams. Is there a difference between eye gels and creams? If so, which one should you use? There is actually a big difference between gels and creams. A gel is much less emollient than a cream. It will contain more water and go on much thinner. Gels quickly dry on the surface of the skin and usually cause a tightening effect. Some manufacturers call this a "lift" effect. In actuality, your skin is being tightened or pulled due to the water evaporating from the gel.

Creams contain more oil than gels; therefore, creams are more emollient or softening. As I have said previously, it is vitally important to keep a lipid (emollient) substance on the lines around the eyes at all times. This is to ensure the under-eye tissue stays soft and pliable, helping to keep the lines less noticeable. Gels will dry out very quickly; creams take a lot longer to actually dry on the skin. If I had to choose between the two, I would pick a cream over a gel.

There are eye gels on the market that contain special ingredients to tackle lines and wrinkles (alpha hydroxy acids, for instance). These are fine to use *underneath* an eye cream, but I would not recommend using these gels alone day to day. However, if you seem to always get puffy eyes using eye creams, try using a gel and see if you have better luck. But for most people and for the easiest approach, stick with eye creams for treating the under-eye area.

How to use eye cream. First, you only want to use a small amount of cream—just enough to smooth on the lines. The more you use, the greater the chances the cream will find its way into your eyes. Sometimes if you apply too much or apply a cream that is heavy, it can cause puffiness when the thin under-eye skin tries to absorb the excess.

You want to be very careful when applying eye cream in order not to stretch or pull this delicate tissue. I always use my ring fingers. Place a small amount of eye cream on one finger and warm it by patting your ring fingers together. Then gently apply to the lines around your eyes. Remember to pat, not rub, the under-eye skin.

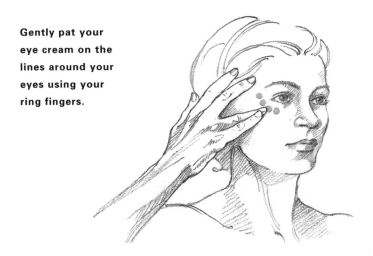

Gently pat your eye cream on the lines around your eyes using your ring fingers.

Clients always ask if they should put eye cream on their eyelids. It's not really necessary. You want eye cream specifically on the lines around the eyes. Too much cream on the lids can cause it to migrate (through warming because the lids are open throughout the day) into the eyes themselves. If you have scaly or excessively dry lids, you can put a small amount of cream there. If you suffer from eczema or some other form of dermatitis, you'll want to seek a dermatologist's care.

When to use eye cream. I like to put eye cream on after moisturizing my face, but you can use it beforehand if you prefer. Either way, you want to use eye cream after cleansing and toning. I also recommend having some on hand to use throughout the day. Because you have no functioning oil glands under the eyes, this tissue tends to dry out quickly, so don't hesitate to reapply as necessary. If you wear make-up, perhaps this won't be possible. But if you don't wear makeup or aren't wearing foundation, feel free to use your eye cream more than twice per day.

Lips

Chapped lips are a problem for a lot of people. If you wear lipstick, you'll want to use anti-chapping products at night before bed and whenever you aren't wearing lipstick. If you have severe problems with chapping, try not wearing lipstick for a few days while using healing lip balms. If your chapped lips clear up, your lipstick may be causing the problem. You may want to switch to a more moisturizing type of lipstick. If you will use healing lip products on a regular basis, most of you will find relief from chapping.

For years I used petroleum-based lip balms, and still my lips stayed very chapped and flaky. I switched brands many times, but never found relief. After a friend brought to my attention the large amounts of petroleum contained in these products, I opted for a healthier type of lip care. Remember, throughout the day you are ingesting (by eating, drinking, and licking off) anything you put on your lips. It may seem minor, but day after day, year after year, the petroleum and dyes in lipsticks and balms add up to consuming a lot of undesirable elements. There are many brands of quality lip care that can be found at most health food stores. My favorite is a nonpetroleum product that smells like citrus. After using a petroleum-free lip balm for over a year now, I hardly need to use one at all.

Try switching to nonpetroleum lip products, and see if that helps you. Some eye creams are made to be used on the lips as well. Personally, I prefer a balm rather than a cream, but you may fare well using your eye cream as a lip treatment.

Using an oil on your lips can also be an effective way to relieve chapping. If you have olive oil in your kitchen, pour some in a small container and dab it on your lips whenever you need to. This will go a long way in helping to keep your lips hydrated and free from chapping.

Quick Tips
- If you don't have time or are too tired to cleanse your skin at night, before you put toothpaste on your toothbrush, put cleanser on your face. Brush your teeth and then you'll have to take the cleanser off.
- If you left your makeup on overnight (shame on you), you'll need to exfoliate (see Chapter 2) to get the imbedded junk out of your pores before you put on another day's makeup. Don't skip this step.
- Although nitrazine papers are expensive, one roll is more than you'll need. You might consider dividing the roll among several friends. The paper strips can be stored in a Ziploc baggie and torn off as needed.
- Put your spray toner in the refrigerator in the summer months so you can enjoy a cool spray of refreshment on your face during a hot summer's day.
- Simplify your cosmetic drawer. Get rid of all those half-filled jars and bottles of potions you never use anymore. I know it's hard to throw those precious products away—they were *expensive!* Use any remaining moisturizers on your body instead of tossing them. Just think how wonderful it will be to open your drawer or cabinet and have less clutter.
- Many sunscreens can be used as your moisturizer. Don't start piling on moisturizer, sunscreen, *and* makeup. It's too much for the pores.

- Buy more than one package of eye cream. Keep an extra one at work, on your nightstand, in your purse, or all of the above. Put it on (sparingly) throughout the day to keep the delicate under-eye tissue soft. It's *that* important.
- Try not to bite off the dry, flaking skin on your chapped lips. This will only perpetuate the problem and give you the potential for open sores where the skin has come off. It's a hard habit to break, but it will help keep your lips from bleeding and give them time to heal.
- I strongly recommend *not* using a magnifying mirror when it comes to looking at your face. Unless you require one to apply makeup, there is no need to make yourself crazy with this unrealistic view of your skin. No one looking at your skin can see what shows up through magnification. Not even you.

The Extras

There are two steps you'll want to add to your Basic 1-2-3 pro-gram on a weekly or biweekly basis that are important for maintaining healthy, problem-free skin. Although they are called "extras," I really consider them to be "essentials." These two steps are exfoliating and using a clay mask. Exfoliating removes the dead cell buildup on your face and leaves your skin soft and smooth. A clay mask deep cleans the pores and soothes your skin. The Basics are your daily maintenance, but The Extras can take your skin one step closer to being its best.

Exfoliation

What is exfoliation? As we age, the regeneration process slows down. This process includes the making and shedding of skin cells. When we're young, our cells are "born." Then they rise to the surface, where they are shed at a very rapid pace. As regeneration starts to slow down (around age 25), the new cells being formed travel to the surface more slowly and tend to pile up on the outside of the skin. The removal of these dead cells is called exfoliation. It allows the younger, newer cells to come up to the surface, making the skin feel softer and look brighter. Exfoliating on a regular basis is one of the most important things you can do for your skin.

Why exfoliate? Dead skin and oil cause plugs to form inside your pores. Keeping the buildup of dead cells to a minimum is important in keeping the pores free from congestion. Not only will exfoliating help maintain clean pores, it will also help your outer skin feel soft and smooth. In addition, exfoliating helps stimulate the circulation, leaving your cells well nourished and healthy. Whenever you exfoliate, you can lift a dull complexion off your face and replace it with smooth skin that reflects light. In other words, exfoliation gives you a healthy glow.

What to use. Scrubs are the most commonly known products for exfoliation. They are a blend of an emollient-based cream or gel with some type of abrasive granules mixed in. These abrasive particles can be organic matter like apricot seeds or tiny polyurethane beads that are synthetic. Because these balls are perfectly round (unlike the irregular shape of seeds), manufactures tout their superiority over seeds. They say the organic seeds may scratch the skin's surface; the rounded balls will not. Be aware that these synthetic beads are so round and *tiny* that they can easily become lodged in your pores and may be difficult to get out if you're not careful.

My experience with these perfectly shaped beads has not been positive. One evening I was experimenting with a new scrub containing the synthetic particles. After rinsing the scrub off my face, I looked in the mirror and discovered one perfect little bead had found a home in a pore on my nose. This foreign object wasn't easy to remove and had I not seen it, it surely would have caused problems. Unless it eventually came out on its own, this little bead could have stretched that particular pore, if not caused something worse down the road.

So if you do end up using a scrub with synthetic particles, just be extra careful. Don't press hard while scrubbing, and closely examine your skin afterwards to make sure you have removed everything from your face. The seed-type scrubs do not usually cause the aforementioned problem, but make sure not to grind the scrub (or anything) into your skin. Although the outer skin is resilient, you still don't want to mash anything into it. As long as you are not sensitive and you use one with care, it is doubtful you can harm your skin (by scratching the surface) with a scrub.

Scrubs should not be used on problem skin or red, irritated skin. If you have acne, scrubs are definitely *out*. The abrasive particles in a scrub can easily open up any infected areas, allowing bacteria to spread, not to mention the irritation a scrub will cause on these sensitive places. A simple rule of thumb is if your skin is red (for whatever reason), don't use a scrub.

Scrubs are excellent for stimulating blood circulation, and this heightened blood flow helps to nourish skin cells. However, scrubs do a minimal job of exfoliating. They just don't get rid of a lot of dead skin. Additionally, after you rinse the scrub off and pat your skin dry with a towel, you may experience a feeling of dryness. This is actually dehydration. You have not only removed some dead cells, but all the oil and water from your skin as well. Unfortunately, this can leave your skin feeling depleted. This is one reason I prefer a gel-type gommage for exfoliating, which is discussed later in this section. These products *add* moisture to the skin through the gel substance instead of removing it like a scrub can.

Papaya enzyme peels are another way to exfoliate. They are a little more effective than a scrub in terms of exfoliation. You generally won't have any problems with irritation since these enzyme peels don't contain granules. The enzymes help to decompose skin cells as well as increase circulation. Typically you apply the peel to your entire face like a mask. As it dries, the product is rubbed off (gently), helping to remove any dead cell buildup on the surface of your skin.

The best and most effective thing to use when exfoliating is a gommage, which is a nonabrasive, gel-type peel. These are harder to find, but they do exist. Rather than using abrasive particles like a scrub, a gommage has a hydrating gel base that gives it a deep moisturizing effect. By massaging this soft peel into your skin (increasing circulation), the gel adheres to your outer dead cells. As the product dries, eraser-like flakes start to appear. These flakes signal the gommage is lifting off surface cells. (In French, *gommer* means to erase.) This will leave your skin feeling very smooth and refined without any irritation from seeds or granules like those found in scrubs. A gel exfoliator is perfect for problem or acne skin because it lessens the potential for opening any lesions or irritating already sensitive skin. Gel exfoliators can also be used around the eyes. This skin needs exfoliation just like the rest of your face. Due to the delicate nature of the under-eye tissue, you never want to use an abrasive scrub there. When using a gommage or anything around or under your eyes, never rub or get aggressive with your skin.

How to exfoliate. Basically, you just follow the directions given for the product you are using. You want to exfoliate your face as well as your neck. I always exfoliate the tops of my hands as well. When you're applying either a scrub or gommage, you want to use light, circular movements—never pulling or digging into the skin. Scrubs always need to be used on *wet* skin. Gommage or enzyme peels are usually applied to dry skin. Whether using a scrub or a gel peel, never use too much pressure—just enough to get the job done. Your skin is resilient, but it is delicate at the same time. Constant rubbing and pulling can affect the elasticity in the long term.

Be careful when using a scrub around your ears not to get any product into the actual ear canal. You can gently scrub behind and in front of your ears, but don't intentionally put scrub inside your ears.

When to exfoliate. Depending on what you're using, you should exfoliate at least once a week. The more you exfoliate, the smoother and healthier your skin will look and feel. This, of course, is assuming you have found an exfoliator that works well for your particular skin. Use a scrub or gommage after cleansing and before moisturizing. (If you plan to use a clay mask, discussed in the next section, exfoliate prior to masking.) If you look in the mirror and wish you could have a facial (or feel you need one), it's a good time to exfoliate. After exfoliating, use Step 2: Toner, then Step 3: Moisturizer (and eye cream), and you're finished.

Quick Tips

- Always use scrubs on wet skin. Used dry, they can drag and pull your skin.
- Don't use scrubs as your cleanser. They don't have the ingredients to break down oil like a cleanser does. Use scrubs to exfoliate dead cells and stimulate circulation.
- If your scrub feels irritating, add it to your cleanser and gently go over your face and neck. If the scrub still irritates your skin, use it on your body or simply throw it away.

- Exfoliating prior to a special occasion will have a twofold benefit for your skin. First, it will exfoliate dead cells, making the surface smoother, helping your makeup go on better. It will also stimulate circulation, making your skin look luminous.
- Using your facial scrub in the shower will help lessen the mess when it comes time to rinse your face.

Clay Mask

What is a clay mask? A clay mask is a deep-cleansing treatment for your pores. It is a mixture of different clays in an emollient or creamy base. The mask usually has a thick consistency and may be brown, green, white, or even blue. Clay is stimulating and calming, as well as deep cleansing. It is good for all skin types and can even be used on irritated skin. Clay is a contact healer and was used by Native Americans as a poultice (a clay "pack") on wounds to stop bleeding and speed healing. Using a clay mask is another important step in keeping your skin clean, clear, and healthy.

Why use a clay mask? A clay mask will help keep the skin clear and the pores cleaned out, which is of paramount importance. Clay helps lift debris and impurities from the pores with its strong drawing ability. Clay has a stimulating effect on the circulation. This brings in oxygen and nutrients from the blood to feed and nourish skin cells. Clay also has a calming effect. Used on skin that is broken out or couperose (broken capillaries making the skin appear red), it can help to temporarily alleviate the redness, leaving the skin looking radiant. After using a clay mask, your face should be very clean, and the surface should be clear with a healthy glow.

I've read skin care books that discourage the use of clay masks. I suppose this is because the authors haven't come across good masks that are truly effective. But effective clay masks do exist, and they are an essential step in your skin care routine, especially if you have clogged pores or problem skin.

What to use. There are several common names for clay you will see in a mask ingredient list: kaolin, bentonite, French clay, China clay, green clay, and others. When looking for a clay mask, you want to make sure clay is one of the first ingredients. Since ingredients are listed by weight, a mask with a large concentration of clay will have clay listed among the first on the list. There are many masks out on the market that claim to be clay or cleansing masks, but they actually have very little clay in them. And that's a shame because you use them, get little or no results, then think all clay masks must be ineffective. Products found in a salon are usually far superior to grocery or department store varieties. Check with your aesthetician (see Chapter 3/Professional Facials), and keep an eye on the ingredient list. Not all clay masks are created equal, so you may have to experiment before you come up with one that works for you.

How can you tell if your clay mask is effective? Before applying the mask, take a good look at your pores. Then after the mask is rinsed off, do the same check. If you don't notice a significant reduction in the amount of debris in your pores, especially around the nose area or wherever you have the most congestion, the mask is not doing its job. Check the ingredients and make sure it is predominately clay. If not, find a new mask that has a higher concentration of clay.

Although you can get dry clay powder at the health food store and mix it with water, I don't recommend using this on your skin. Even if you don't have sensitive skin, clay with no other ingredients is just too intense and too concentrated. Find a manufactured mask that has a high percentage of clay in it, and use it at least once a week to deep cleanse your pores.

How to use a clay mask. *Never let clay dry on your face.* In fact, you don't really want *anything* to dry on the surface. This will dry out the surface of your skin. It's like taking one step forward, two steps back. Clay doesn't need to dry in order to draw impurities to itself. There are actually cleansing fasts that require you to ingest certain types of clay. Obviously the whole time the clay is in your body, it remains moist, yet it still draws out toxins while it's going through your system. Here, you're just applying clay to your face, but the principle is the same. Clay does not need to dry on the skin in order to draw out superficial debris. This may contradict how you have always been told to use a clay mask, but hopefully it makes sense to you.

On clean, dry skin, apply a thick layer of clay mask over your entire face, avoiding the eye area. *Thick layer* means thick enough so you can't see your skin underneath. A thin application will quickly dry on your skin. Unless your neck is broken out, you don't need to apply clay there. Instead, you can apply a hydrating mask or a thick layer of your moisturizer to include your neck in this treatment. Don't forget to get some clay directly under your chin as well as that place between your jawbone and earlobe. I normally apply the clay right up on my earlobe. This whole little area tends to collect debris, and sometimes blackheads will form. Using a clay mask in these hard-

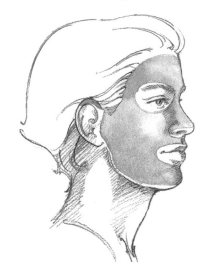

Apply clay mask over your entire face, avoiding the skin directly under your eyes. Be sure to get it all the way over to your ear- lobes and just under your chin.

to-reach areas will lessen the chance of congestion. Leave the mask on for 15 minutes or so. If you don't have 15 minutes but you really need to apply a mask, keep it on for 5 to 10 minutes. Using it even for short amounts of time is better than not using it at all.

After your time is up, rinse the clay off with tepid water, pat your skin dry, use your toner, and moisturize. When it comes time to rinse the mask off, you'll be glad you kept it moist. A dried-on, hardened clay mask is very difficult to remove.

How to keep the mask moist. As I stated earlier, you want to keep the clay mask moist the entire time it's on your face. At your local beauty supply or grocery store, purchase an empty spray bottle (like the kind you put your toner in). Fill it with clean, filtered water. Immediately after you've applied the mask, spray your face thoroughly with the water. After five minutes or so, you'll feel the mask starting to dry (especially around the periphery where the mask is most thin), so grab your bottle and spray your face again. During the 15 minutes you have the mask on, you will probably spray 3 or 4 times—whatever it takes to keep the clay moist.

Where to use a clay mask. If you are a bath-type person, this is a good place to do a clay mask. Put the clay on your clean, dry face, then grab your spray bottle and hop into the tub. Relax, enjoy, and every so often spray your face. I don't recommend splashing the bathwater on your face, especially if you have used any bath products in the water. This can really irritate your skin.

Using a clay mask in a steam room is the perfect marriage of protection and cleansing. The steam is great for stimulating the circulation, but remember the capillaries are very fragile and cannot withstand the intense heat in a steam room. Putting a clay mask on your face creates an occlusive, protective barrier between your skin and the hot steam. And since the clay will stay perfectly moist in this environment, it is an ideal place to use your mask. Also note that if you find yourself in a steam room without a clay mask handy, I highly recommend wetting a few paper towels and putting them over your face while steaming. The heat is just too intense for your face and can really cause a good deal of capillary damage if you frequent steam rooms "unprotected." Usually the paper towels at a gym are stiff enough (even when wet) to make a good cover for your face.

When to use a clay mask. Clay can be used as often as desired. If you have normal to oily skin, blackheads, or any congestion, you will want to use clay at least once a week to keep the pores cleaned out. If you have problem skin, you'll want to mask several times per week. And finally, even true-dry skin can benefit from using a clay mask. Oil-deficient skin doesn't require the same deep cleansing as does an oilier skin type, but you can still derive many benefits from using a clay mask once every week or two.

It's best to mask *after* exfoliating if you're using them together. Exfoliation will help get rid of excess dead skin as well as superficial debris in the pores. The clay mask further deep cleans the pores along with helping to soothe and calm the surface. Exfoliating and using a clay mask can be done in tandem, once a week (or more) as a mini, at-home facial. They do not need to be done together, but it's nice to do both if you have the time. Exfoliate, run a bath, put the clay mask on, hop in, and relax. After removing the mask, use your toner and moisturizer along with eye cream. For more details, see At-Home Facials in the next section.

Quick Tips
- Dot the clay mask on blemishes after your evening 1-2-3 routine and leave on overnight. Clay will help to diminish (but not totally clear) the spots.

- If you're short on time and need to mask, five minutes before your morning shower apply a clay mask. Jump into the shower, and the mask will stay moist from the steam. Remove it at the end of your shower, then use your toner and moisturizer (Steps 2 & 3).

At-Home Facials

An at-home facial is an attempt to simulate the benefits of a professional facial in the comfort (and convenience) of your own home. Like giving yourself a massage, nothing takes the place of having someone else do all the work for you, but you can duplicate many of the steps of a facial yourself, which will benefit your skin as well as give you an overall feeling of relaxation.

An at-home facial incorporates exfoliating, using a clay mask, and relaxing. To accomplish this, you'll need about half an hour or so. You can embellish on my suggestions or tailor them to your particular schedule. If you are too busy to slow down completely, you can just exfoliate and mask, then be on your way. But taking a few minutes out of a hectic day to relax and unwind sure feels good.

Make your bathroom a temporary relaxation sanctuary. Fill the room with candles, draw an aromatic bath, and listen to relaxing music to ease the stresses of the day from your body. If you're not a bath-type person, find a room in your house where you can relax—undisturbed—for 15 minutes or so. It would also be nice to have soothing music to assist you into a calm, meditative state.

If you are a bath person, you are well aware of the healing powers of taking a relaxing soak. It is a restorative pleasure. Baths give you a moment to slow down and take some time for you. The wet heat is one of the best ways to soothe aching muscles. I like to use bath salts because they are aromatic (a bath filled with bath salts is like incense for your home) and can help to relieve muscle aches as well as stimulate circulation. Bath oils are also aromatic and will help to moisturize rough, dry skin while you bathe. (See Chapter 11/Moisturizing.)

Even if you don't have a lot of time to luxuriate in the tub, try to find at least 15 minutes one day a week. Tell your husband and the kids you are locking yourself in the bathroom, and short of an emergency, you are not available. (I jokingly told a client to get a "Do Not Disturb" sign for her bathroom door. Maybe it's not such a bad idea!) Putting aside time for *you* gives you more energy to give to others. It's a simple principle, although not always so easy to implement.

To begin your at-home facial, you'll want to thoroughly wash your face. Next, use your exfoliator of choice. Be sure to take a little extra time and get all the nooks and crannies well exfoliated. You might want to read over Chapter 12 (The Forgotten Places) describing the areas we sometimes neglect. Finally, apply the clay mask. Have your water mister handy to keep the mask moist, go to your peaceful place (either your quiet room or bathtub), and relax. Breathe in the calmness in the air and exhale all the stress that has built up in your body. Let the world go by without worrying about it.

When your time is up, remove the clay mask at your sink—not with the bath water. Another alternative would be to shower after your bath and remove the mask this way. Once the clay is rinsed off, use your toner (Step 2) and moisturizer (Step 3). Don't forget eye cream as well.

After your bath, be sure to moisturize your body. Use this time to treat your *whole* body, not just your face. If you're up for it, read Chapter 11 for more ideas on taking care of the skin on your body.

An at-home facial can be done on the road or in your home, whenever you need a mini-break from a stressful day. It may seem impossible to take time out for yourself, but once you do you will know it *is* possible. At-home facials can benefit you on several levels just like a professional facial can. Enjoy your treatment and know you are helping yourself in many ways, not just your skin.

Advanced steps. Here are a few advanced techniques for those of you who want to go the extra mile. These are not necessary to do in order to get the full benefits from an at-home facial. They are simply additional steps for the person who wants to take the extra time.

1. Use moisturizer underneath your clay mask. With the mask lying on top, it will help to infuse the cream deep into your skin, giving you an extra dose of hydration. Cleanse your skin, exfoliate, and then before applying the clay mask put on a medium to thick layer of your favorite moisturizing cream. Apply your clay mask, spraying it with water intermittently to keep it moist as mentioned earlier. Leave it on for 15 minutes, then remove the mask by splash-rinsing with tepid water. Use your toner (Step 2) and moisturizer (Step 3).

2. Place soothing eye pads over your eyes and relax to treat the eye area during your at-home facial. One way to do this is to steep chamomile tea (or any other relaxing, soothing herb) for several hours. Place the concentrated tea in the refrigerator to cool (perhaps the night before you are planning your facial). Then when you're ready to lie down and relax with the clay mask on in your quiet room or bathtub, soak two cotton pads in the cooled tea and place them over your eyes. Lie back and relax, keeping the mask moist by misting with your spray bottle. When your mask is ready to come off, remove the eye pads, splash-rinse, then tone and hydrate with your moisturizer.

Ponds™ came out with cucumber eye pads that are fun and easy to use although they are a bit pricey. They have a high percentage of cucumber extract and other soothing ingredients in them. They even look like cucumbers. If you like to use eye pads, these are a fun alternative.

Another option is to wet a couple of round eye pads, then spray a small amount of your toner on them. Squeeze most of the moisture out, and then place the pads over your eyes. The water will dilute your toner, making soothing eye pads that are inexpensive, readily available, and easy to use.

3. Apply a thick layer of eye cream before you put the pads on for extra treatment of the eyes. Or if you want to skip eye pads altogether, simply put a thick layer of eye cream on, lie back, and relax. This under-eye skin needs special treatment too.

4. Include your neck as well as treating the skin around your eyes. If you have a special hydrating mask, this would be a good time to use it. After the clay is on your face, apply a thick layer of hydrating mask to your entire neck area. If you don't have a specialized hydrating mask, just use a thick layer of your moisturizer. Either one will do a good job of moisturizing this forgotten area.

A word about food as products. I'm not a fan of using home-made products on your face. If these kitchen products are good enough to eat, then you should eat them, not put them topically on your skin. Your body can utilize the nutrients in food much more readily than your skin can. Homemade products can be too intense and concentrated for a lot of skins. But if you feel the need to blend something up for your face, go right ahead. It probably won't be harmful to your skin although most likely it will be of little help. If you feel any irritation, immediately remove the homemade product and reach for a manufactured one next time.

Quick Tips
- Music can have a therapeutic and relaxing effect after a stressful day. If you aren't sleeping well, try playing a meditation tape while lying in bed. This type of music has a monotone without a lot of crescendo. It is ideal to help your mind stop working so hard,

which is usually what is keeping you up. I have made many tapes for clients who were either under stress or just having trouble getting to sleep from time to time. Some artists and titles are listed in the Suggested Listening section at the end of this chapter.

- I also recommend this type of music for a baby who is having trouble sleeping. My clients are quite relieved to find these soothing tones help lull their babes to sleep.
- To involve your kids and perhaps give them a better understanding of your quiet time, have them draw or paint a creative Do Not Disturb sign for you to hang on the bathroom door.
- I like to use relaxation time in the bath to say my daily affirmations (prayers). All distractions are gone, and I can concentrate on the words I am reciting. (I do this in the shower too.)
- If you travel, packing an inflatable bath pillow can help you enjoy your bath time while on the road. They are inexpensive (usually under $5) and won't take up much space in your travel bag.

Suggested Listening

Angel Love by Aeoliah (Helios Music 800-900-5997)
Aura Sound I and *Aura Sound II* by William Aura
    (Higher Octave Music)
Eastern Peace, Inner Peace, and *Spectrum Suite* by Stephen Halpern
    (Open Channel Sound Co./BMI)
Fragrances of a Dream and *Velvet Dreams* by Daniel Kolbialka
    (Li-Sem Enterprises, Inc.)
Inside the Cathedral, Inside the Taj Mahal, and *Music* by Paul Horn
    (CBS Records, Inc.)
Meditation Healing Music by Fumio (BIWA USA)
Musical Massage (The Relaxation Company)
Quiet Music 1,2, and *3* by Steven Roach (Fortuna Records)

3

Professional Facials

Getting a facial means different things to different people. For some it is a conditioning treatment to maintain their already healthy skin. For others it is a necessary step for keeping their skin trouble-free. Truly, you can benefit from a facial no matter what condition your skin is in. Just like getting your teeth cleaned at the dentist, a facial gets rid of imbedded debris and deep cleans the pores. These treatments will also superhydrate your outer skin and can go a long way in helping your whole body relax, if only for that hour. Although styles of treatment vary from place to place, I have listed some of the many advantages of getting a professional facial.

Deep cleansing. Initially your face is washed with gentle surface cleansers before it is analyzed with the aid of a magnifying lamp to determine the course of treatment. A procedure known as extraction, where blackheads and whiteheads are carefully removed from the pores manually, is performed when necessary and is an integral part of the deep-cleansing process. Toward the end of the facial, a clay mask is commonly used to further cleanse the pores by lifting out surface debris. No matter what kind of facial you receive, your skin should come out very clean and the pores free from debris.

Exfoliation. This is the sloughing off or removal of outer, dead cells, which leaves the texture of your skin smoother and more refined. It is dead skin and oil that clog the pores, so keeping the surface free from a buildup of dead cells helps fight congestion and enables your skin to retain moisture, making it feel smoother. Different salons incorporate different procedures, but nearly every facial will include some form of exfoliation.

Hydration. Throughout the facial, many nourishing and moisturizing creams are massaged into the skin. Sometimes ampoules (vials containing concentrated extracts or oils) are applied as well. All skin can utilize the benefits of deep hydration. Even oily and problem skin needs to be well hydrated, making the texture feel smoother and the skin look healthier in general.

Relaxation. Listed last, but certainly not least, the relaxation benefits you receive from having a facial are undeniable. We all have a lot of stress in our busy lives, and it's important to balance this out with what I call "anti-stress activities." Whether you're relaxing in a tub full of bubbles or finding quiet time to read a book, taking time to balance out the stress in your life is the key to health and well-being. A facial offers you fantastic relaxation benefits. In fact, many people are surprised at how relaxing facials really are. Getting a facial truly is a great escape, a haven where no one can find you. When my clients walk through the door to my office, they instantly start to relax. I'm not pulling teeth here. They know they can let the stresses of the day go, even if it's just for an hour. Relaxation is a hidden benefit that should not be overlooked when considering having a facial.

When you leave the treatment room, your skin should be very clean, well exfoliated, superhydrated, and smooth to the touch and have a healthy, well-nourished glow. Allow yourself an escape once in a while with a wonderfully relaxing facial—for your health.

How Often?

Once a month is a common recommendation for getting regular facials. Every 28 days or so (sometimes a bit longer if you're older), your skin cells regenerate. New cells are coming up to the surface and flattening out to form the uppermost part of the epidermis, while older cells are being shed. When you have a facial once a month, you are supplying the newly forming cells with good nutrition through increased blood circulation as well as getting rid of dead cells ready to come off. A facial in effect enhances the natural life, death, and removal of skin cells.

Having a facial more often, once a week for instance, would be even more beneficial for your skin. But few people have the time or the money to do this. If I could, I would have a facial once a week and a massage every day. But for most people (myself included), this is a fantasy. My point is, more often is always better than less often when getting regular facials. And regularity is the key word. Rather than having a treatment once a week for a few months and then not seeing the inside of a salon for nine months, getting a facial less often (every four to eight weeks), but *consistently*, will yield the best results. You will receive immediate short-term benefits from a single facial treatment, but only by having regular, consecutive facials will you experience long-term results.

Another consideration is the condition of your skin. People with problem skin will want to have facials as often as possible to help keep their skin on the road to recovery. Skin that is broken out can really experience good results from professional treatments. Those of you with few or no problems will benefit from regular, monthly facials as well. Everyone needs extra exfoliation, more hydration, and deep cleaning no matter the type or condition of the skin. I can definitely tell a difference in a client who has had monthly facials over a period of several years. There is a certain clarity and softness to her skin that is unmistakable. The lines are less noticeable, and her skin, quite simply, looks healthy. Usually she has a good understanding of her skin and knows the value of consistent care.

The importance of professional treatments cannot be overemphasized, but without daily at-home care, professional facials can only take you so far. Optimum results occur when incorporating good skin care habits at home as well as facials in a salon. Time and money usually dictate how often you can have a professional treatment. First spend your money on good at-home products (since you'll be affecting your skin on a daily basis), then try to have a facial every four weeks. If this is not possible, six to eight weeks would be my next recommendation. Even getting a facial seasonally will do a lot to help prepare your skin for whatever changes the weather will bring.

Where To Look

Finding a good professional facial involves two key elements. First, you need to find a qualified aesthetician (a person licensed to perform facials). Then you want to find someone who uses quality products. Both the aesthetician and the product need to be good for the facial to be worth your time and money. You may have to go through some trial and error before you find the perfect facial for you.

The easiest way to find someone who is good at her craft is through a friend's referral. You want suggestions from someone who has had a lot of facials, a person whose opinion you respect. If your friends don't get them, ask if someone they know can steer you to a good place for a facial. If you've just moved to a new town, ask everyone you meet for a referral, and if the same name keeps coming up, you can start there. (My entire business is built from referrals. It's the best advertising there is.) If you can't get a referral, go to the Yellow Pages and start calling salons.

When a client moves out of town, I call around to salons in her area to gather information that will help me determine where she might find a good facial. I recommend doing this yourself if you don't know where to go. Believe it or not, these initial calls will tell you a lot. Keep in mind, you're looking for a *professional*. Ask to speak to the aesthetician if she's available. If not, you'll have to settle for whoever can answer your questions. Here's what to ask:

1. What type of business is it? Is it a full-service salon with hair, nails, and massage, or exclusively skin care? Is it a salon with several aestheticians or an individual running her own business? The individual business owner is more likely to provide the most private environment. She may, however, be leasing space within a large salon, so if size matters to you, be sure and ask. Large salons tend to be less private, with many people coming in and out of them all day long. Some people like more privacy; others enjoy the energy of a busy salon.

2. Which products does the salon use? If you're not familiar with the products they use, don't worry. Eventually you'll have firsthand experience with different product lines and can make an educated decision about their effectiveness with your particular skin. If you know the products they use, you may or may not need to ask further questions. **Are samples available?** I rarely sell products to a first-time client. Not that I won't, but I prefer to send my client home with samples so she can determine, in the privacy and comfort of her own home, if they are worth the investment. High-quality, effective products will sell themselves without high-pressure sales tactics. If you can't sample the product (and even if you can), be clear about the salon's return policy before you decide to buy.

3. How long has the aesthetician worked there? Is she new? Has she worked in five different places in the past two years? If she's worked there a long time, at least you know she's stable and probably has a large and satisfied clientele. If you are just going for an occasional facial, these particular questions aren't going to be very important to you. But if you are looking for a salon or an aesthetician to get regular facials from, keep this in mind: you are looking to build a relationship. The aesthetician's personality, her knowledge about skin care, her reliability, stability, etc., are all going to be important qualities to look for. If she tends to move around a lot, and you like her facials, you may find yourself moving around with her. This may not necessarily be a negative, although it could get quite inconvenient for you.

4. How long has she been an aesthetician? The first few years after skin care school are when your education truly begins. Right after school and without practical experience, you simply don't know as much as you will in later years. A novice aesthetician is *not* what you are looking for. **Does she use the product herself?** You'd be surprised how many people don't use the products they sell. That's a very bad sign. The skill of the aesthetician plus her commitment to a product are what make a facial great.

5. How long is the facial? The person you speak to may ask you, "Which one?" I'll tell you right now I'm not a fan of "menus" when it comes to facials, yet most salons will have one. In my own business, I have one facial that includes everything possible for each individual's skin to be its best. I do not add costly steps while "en route," nor do I believe the client should be deciding what her skin needs. It's not a restaurant where you order what you want; it's a treatment based on a professional analysis of what's going on with your skin. The aesthetician should decide the course of treatment for the client, not the other way around. Facials usually last from one to one and a half hours. Anything less than an hour may not be enough time to have quality work done.

6. Does the salon use machines? Machines are very common, and I have listed those most often used in facials. The salon you go to may employ all or none of them. Keep in mind machines lack the sensitivity of human contact. Studies show the tremendous healing benefits of touch. It calms the nervous system, and gives you, the client, a sense of connection to the aesthetician. If machines are used every step of the way, I'd keep calling around.

Steam. This is the most widely used piece of machinery. Almost every facial offers steam. The mist superficially hydrates the outer skin and softens debris held in the pores, ideally making extractions easier. I have found, however, that once the steam is removed, the debris inside the pores hardens, making extractions *more* difficult. The heat from the steam stimulates circulation, which helps to nourish the cells, although the heat may become too intense for several skin conditions. If you have acne, capillary damage, redness, or sensitive skin, you are *not* a good candidate for steam. In fact, you should avoid it. If you find yourself in a treatment where steam is used, and you have one of these skin conditions, ask the aesthetician to either move the steam farther from your face or do away with it all together. Steam is a superfluous step in many ways, but most facials incorporate it. A beneficial time to utilize the steam machine is during the clay mask. Request that it be used then in order to keep the clay moist. Beware, they may balk at this suggestion, but explain that you don't want the clay to dry on your face or the steam on your bare skin. (See Chapter 2/How to use a clay mask.)

Brush machine. The brush machine eliminates dead surface cells by using a rotating brush attached to a motorized unit. The brushes spin at various speeds, come in different textures, and are generally made of goat hair. One problem I have with this machine is sanitation. The brushes are used on everyone who has been to that salon for a facial. Of course they are properly sanitized (you hope), but how long has a particular brush been in use? This machine should never be used on acne, red, or sensitive skin. It should never be used on skin with broken capillaries. It's not the worst thing in the world, but at the very least, human touch is once again replaced by a machine.

Your choices for exfoliation in a facial are sometimes limited to the brush machine or a scrub. Neither is terribly effective, but unless the product line the salon uses has other options for exfoliation, you may be faced with this machine. Most salons now include mild to strong acid peels within the facial.

The vacuum. Yes, that's right—a *vacuum*. I can't believe these are still used today, but they are. In case you come across the vacuum in a facial, just say "NO!" Its purpose is to suction out imbedded dirt and debris from the pores. Unfortunately, it can cause capillary damage due to the suction and is very ineffective at cleaning out the pores. A vacuum should be used on a floor, not on your face.

Galvanic current. This machine uses a low-level current and two terminals, or poles. One pole is positively charged; the other is negatively charged. Sometimes these poles are called "active" and "indifferent." The client holds the negative or indifferent pole, and the active pole is placed on the skin, creating a circuit. The purpose of this machine is to make products penetrate deeper into the skin as well as soften tissue and stimulate circulation. It is my contention that products applied manually penetrate far enough into the skin without the need to incorporate electrically charged machines. I find these devices disruptive to the natural flow of the facial. They aren't used very often, although some salons subscribe to the benefits of machines and will employ galvanic current.

High-frequency. This machine uses infrared light that is either violet or orange-red. The light is directed through a glass electrode that is in turn applied to the skin. (When the machine is turned on, it sounds a bit like Dr. Frankenstein's laboratory.) The uses for a high-frequency machine are to stimulate circulation, warm the surface of the skin, as well as to disinfect the skin. The client's entire face is gone over with a mushroom-shaped electrode, or individual blemishes can be zapped by lifting the electrode off the skin just over the problem spot. This lifting causes a slight shock or spark that has a concentrated, germicidal effect, destroying bacteria. High-frequency is also used to aid in the penetration of products. Here again, there is only so far a product can go into the skin. I don't feel the need to use a machine to penetrate products when a pair of hands can do the job. Manually applying products soothes the client with human touch as well.

Many skin care salons utilize the high-frequency machine, so you will probably come in contact with it. You might want to give it a try to see if you enjoy this form of treatment. I don't use any machines in my facial. I prefer to use my hands and let the products do their magic. Machines leave me cold, and stimulating someone's skin this way doesn't feel right to me. Earlier in my career I had access to a high-frequency machine. I rarely used it because I felt it was doing little to improve my clients' skin and added a strange, cold indifference to the facial. Employing foreign objects with peculiar, electrical noises in place of the soothing nature of human touch didn't create the relaxing environment I wanted to provide for my clients.

Oxygen facials. These treatments usually combine products with special oxygen-related ingredients, along with pure oxygen applied directly to the skin. The products supposedly reduce the function of the skin so the oxygen can penetrate through the skin's barrier. Then a blast of oxygen from a tank is applied to your face, and voila—your skin miraculously absorbs this added oxygen! Actually, most doctors agree that although this is surely a harmless treatment, you cannot make oxygen penetrate into the skin this way.

Having a blast of oxygen directed at your face may feel good and may do wonders for your circulation, but the oxygen carried in your blood is what is feeding and nourishing the skin—from the inside out. There are many people, many *professionals*, who may disagree with me. There are also a lot of people making money selling these kinds of facials. I have a very different approach to skin care. It rarely, if ever, incorporates the latest trends or fads that are presented to the public. Perhaps mine is an old-fashioned approach. I don't, however, see any great improvements in skin after having trendy treatments (such as oxygen facials) or using the latest miracle product. If you're curious about this or any other procedure or skin treatment, check it out and see for yourself whether or not you receive the results that are promised. Oxygen facials tend to be quite expensive, so be forewarned.

And oxygen bars? These booths or bars administer large amounts of oxygen, which is supposed to be purifying. The truth is, your body breathes in oxygen and exhales carbon dioxide perfectly without any help. Trust your body and seek to cleanse and purify it through proven, effective means such as diet and exercise.

Comedone extractor. This is a metal instrument that looks similar to a knitting needle. It has a small, donut-shaped hole at one end. As the hole encircles the blackhead and pressure is applied, the extractor helps to drive debris out of the blackhead. As the name implies, it is to be used on comedones, the technical term for blackheads. Used on closed pores, a comedone extractor could lead to disaster. I highly discourage letting anyone use one of these instruments on you. The aesthetician has little or no sense of how much pressure she is applying. At the very least, this can cause capillary damage, not to mention the insensitivity of unyielding metal on your face. I would *never* use one of these in a treatment or even on my own skin.

Lancets. A lancet is a disposable pin or needle-like implement originally designed for diabetics to prick a finger in order to draw blood and test their blood sugar levels. Lancets are used in facials to make a tiny opening in a closed pore or pustule so the debris can gently be nudged out through the opening. Not to fear, a lancet is not used to dig into the blemish. In the hands of a skilled aesthetician, it can be an effective tool to help with extractions.

7. What about extractions? I am wary of a place that doesn't provide this service. I've heard more than one story of clients in desperate need of extractions who find themselves in a salon that refuses to do them. Conversely, I know many clients who truly needed few or no extractions and were "mashed" needlessly. Once again, the skill of the aesthetician comes into play. But an aesthetician or a salon with a "no extractions" policy is saying that they are unwilling to treat all skin conditions. They will not be able to give you what you potentially need. If you know you need extractions, asking this question will quickly eliminate any salon that refuses to do them. If you positively don't need extractions, or you simply abhor extractions and don't want them done, then going to a salon that doesn't provide that service won't be a problem for you.

8. How much does the facial cost? Prices vary, so you'll want to call around and know the going rate for facials in your area, so there are no surprises. If one facial is a lot more expensive than the next, you'll want to find out why. Price is another area where menus come into play. And again, this is another reason I don't like them. I believe each person should get a whole and complete facial dictated by his or her individual needs. One facial may cost less than another, but perhaps you won't get everything your skin needs for the lesser price. **Is the price all-inclusive or can extras be added?** Unfortunately I have heard many stories of clients who went in to get a $65 facial and came out paying $90 or more. Ouch! There is a little trick you'll want to watch out for, and it goes something like this: you go into the salon you've chosen expecting a $65 facial. But as the aesthetician works on you, she keeps mentioning how dehydrated you are or repeatedly noting some other problem. "You need deep exfoliation," she says. And you agree. Then when you get your bill, you may be surprised to find you agreed to an extra $20 or $30 service! Make sure to ask if the facial includes everything or if exfoliation, masks, ampoules, etc., are an extra charge. If some of these are not included, you still may want to add them, but certainly you want to know the cost beforehand. A facial, in my opinion, should include everything needed for that client during each treatment without extra charges being tacked on.

9. What will my skin look like afterwards? Your skin should look radiant. It should be clean, clear, and healthy-looking. Unless you have problem skin that requires a lot of extraction, your skin should not be red, irritated, or feel greasy with excess cream needing to be wiped off. Your skin should look and feel great.

10. Will makeup be applied after the facial? There are two reasons you don't want to apply makeup after a facial. First and foremost, your skin has just been thoroughly cleansed. The last thing you want to do is cover it up with makeup. Second, it is a signal you'll no doubt be in for a big sales pitch. You're a captive audience when someone is applying makeup to you, and it can cause even the strongest resister to cave in. Let your skin have a break from makeup for a while. Perhaps the salon wants to use makeup to hide the work they did in the facial. Remember, your skin should look great afterwards. Why cover it up? You may be going out right after a facial and need to apply some makeup. Go ahead, but don't make it an after-facial habit.

What To Expect

Here are a few explanations of what you might expect when you have a professional facial. This is a mixture of my own experiences of having facials along with what I offer my clients. Your experience will differ here and there. This is just meant to be a general indication of what to look for and expect.

Entering the salon. Is it clean or in disarray? Is it comfortable and inviting? Would you want to come back to this environment on a regular basis?

The greeting. Are you greeted within a reasonable time or are you wandering around waiting to be helped? Is the staff friendly or uninterested? It never ceases to amaze me how few businesses understand the concept of the first impression. It *is* important, and your initial perception of a place will usually be accurate.

The aesthetician. The first thing you want to look at is the skin of the person about to give you a facial. It's not a good sign if she has an excessive amount of breakout. Remember, this is the person about to advise you on how to take care of your skin. Is she wearing a lot of makeup? How can you see her skin if it's covered up? She should not have nails, and no fingernail polish. Don't forget her hands are going to be on your face; nails are a definite no-no. Don't be fooled by a white lab coat. It may give you the impression of a medical environment, but it's really just a white jacket worn over clothes. Lab coats are regulation in a hospital or doctor's office, but they are merely a facade in a salon.

Changing clothes. You will either change in the facial room itself or in a designated dressing room. Either way, you will be left alone to put on a smock that usually is knee-length and leaves your shoulders bare. A gentleman will either take off his shirt and leave his own pants on, or the aesthetician will provide him with gym shorts to change into.

The room. Facial rooms range from small to tiny. Don't expect a lot of space. I have been in facial rooms that barely allowed for the aesthetician to sit at the head of the facial chair. Most have a sink and a counter for products. Trolleys on rollers are often used to hold supplies within easy access of the technician. The room should be clean and orderly without a lot of clutter. Sometimes there are candles lit for atmosphere and licenses hanging on the walls. Since you are going to be lying down with your eyes closed for most of the treatment, as long as the room is clean, not much else matters.

The chair. Facial chairs vary in size, shape, and design. Although termed *chairs*, they are actually beds that you lie on in order to receive the facial treatment. Many look like upright chairs at first. Then as you sit down, the chair is unfolded into a bed and you are then lying down.

Hopefully the chair will be comfortable; unfortunately not all are. If it isn't, you may be forced to find another salon. Don't forget, you'll be lying in this chair for at least one hour, which might become excruciating if you're not comfortable. If you think something can be done to make it more comfortable (using a rolled-up towel under your knees, for instance), make your requests known. The aesthetician can't read your mind, so don't be shy about communicating your needs. How accommodating she is will tell you a lot.

Preparing you, the client. You will climb into the facial chair, which will be covered with sheets and a blanket or two. I'm very cold-natured, so no matter how many layers are offered, I usually need an additional blanket. In the winter, I have an electric blanket that I cover my clients with. Don't hesitate to ask for more warmth, or for the blankets to be removed if you're too hot. The key is for you to be comfortable. Remember, you're paying for this. Also note that it's a good idea before climbing into the chair and starting an hour-long treatment to use the bathroom, so you won't have to get up in the middle of the facial.

Music. Sound is unfortunately disregarded by a lot of salons, yet music is very important to the overall mood of the room. Some places have individual CD or tape players for each room; others have music piped in from a central location. Some salons I've been to had either no music or a radio on instead. Calm, soothing music can help you nod off or at least feel relaxed. A lack of background noise makes you focus on all the little sounds the aesthetician is making, including her breathing. And a radio, unless requested by the client, has no place in a facial. If you find there isn't music in the room where you're having a facial, request some and see what happens. Maybe they just forgot to turn it on.

Ask questions. I have a client who went to get facials for over ten years with one particular aesthetician. My client never knew what product was being used on her skin and the aesthetician never talked to her about home-care products or even skin care in general. I frequently hear about aestheticians who are not terribly responsible as far as helping clients with their skin. Although it really is the aesthetician's job to explain things to you, I also feel it is up to you to ask questions if you feel unsure about what is being done in the facial as well as what your at-home program should be.

In case the aesthetician you go to doesn't volunteer much information, here are some good questions to ask that will help you determine (a) things about your skin and (b) if she is knowledgeable and qualified in her field.

- How would you classify my skin? Or, what is my skin type?
- Is my skin clean? Are my pores congested?
- Am I dehydrated?
- Do you see sun damage? Capillary damage?
- Do you see any unusual moles?
- Is there anything I'm not doing I should be doing? Or vice versa?
- Tell me about the products you use. What makes them so special?
- What should my basic, daily skin care routine consist of?

I feel that during your first facial, the aesthetician should explain what is being done, why it's being done, and what it will do to your skin. In my own experience of getting facials and in my clients' experiences, this is rarely done. I recommend telling the aesthetician you are very interested in what she is doing and asking if she would please explain each step as she goes so you can have a better understanding of her facial procedures. If she describes what she's doing but not why, ask questions. If what she says doesn't make sense, ask if she can explain it in a different way. A good aesthetician will be able to communicate with you without using a lot of skin care jargon. Keep in mind, this isn't rocket science—something a lot of aestheticians in white lab coats may want you to believe.

When looking for an aesthetician, you want someone with a point of view similar to your own. If you haven't really formulated a viewpoint on skin care, look for someone who says things that make sense to you—common sense. Unfortunately, using verbose, aesthetic, or pseudo-medical jargon seems to be a popular way to communicate with clients. If you don't understand what your aesthetician is talking about, ask questions. Her job is not to make you feel inferior or stupid for being inquisitive, but to help you understand your skin.

All the questions are really just to get you familiar with the procedure and with the person giving you the treatment. After the first facial, most of your questions will have been answered, and in subsequent treatments you can lie there in silence while the facial is being performed. And some of you may simply want to enjoy your facial (even the first one) and not ask any questions. In either case, just lie back, enjoy, and reap the benefits of a relaxing facial.

A word about spas. I worked in a spa for nearly seven years, and I am familiar with how they operate. Don't be fooled or convinced of the quality of a facility merely by their advertisements. The physical structure alone does not make a spa great. It is the people working there that will have the biggest impact on you and will make the biggest difference in the quality of your experience. A spa may hold on to a good review or reputation for years, long after the staff that made it great has left.

Many of my clients have frequented spas here in the U.S. as well as traveled to spas all over the world. Sometimes they're great; sometimes they are a disappointment. Both experiences will cost you the same. There is not enough space in this book to detail how to choose a spa, but one important piece of advice would be to ask a lot of questions. Call first and get the lowdown on the staff and what treatments are offered. It will be hit or miss as to getting good treatments, but at least you can go in knowing what products they use in their facial and body treatments and how long the staff has been there. Personal experience, as always, will be your greatest teacher. Just like finding a good facial, a referral will go a long way in helping you choose a good spa.

Suggested Reading

Healthy Escapes by Bernard Burt (New York: Fodor's Travel Publications, Inc., 1998) includes spas, fitness resorts, and cruises.

Spa Finders Guide to Spa Vacations At Home & Abroad by Jeffrey Joseph (New York: John Wiley & Sons, Inc., 1990). Although it's an older publication, this well-designed book is helpful for finding the perfect spa for you.

Stern's Guide to the Greatest Resorts of the World by Steven B. Stern (Gretna, Louisiana: Pelican Publishing Company, 1998) contains color photographs as well as descriptions of 100 of the best resorts around the world.

Vacations That Can Change Your Life by Ellen Lederman (Naperville, Illinois: Sourcebooks, Inc., 1998) is an unusual book focusing not so much on traditional luxury spa vacations but experiences for the mind, body, and spirit. I include it here because I think it's a wonderful book.

Skin Types

I have read several books that recommend how to determine your skin type. The suggestion is usually to wash your face and leave it bare (don't tone or moisturize) for 30 minutes. Then take a Kleenex and press it to your face, and wherever there is oil left on the tissue is where you have oily skin. I have tried this method and found it to be fairly inaccurate. The best way to find oil on your skin is to simply look. In fact, looking for oiliness or a lack of oil is the number one factor for determining your skin type. Next, you'll want to consider dehydration as well as sensitivity. Problems such as breakout and acne are addressed in Chapter 5.

When analyzing a new client's skin, the first thing I look for is how much oil is being emitted—too much, not enough? Are the pores filled up with oil or too small to see? Then, where are the pores congested? Is it mostly on the nose, forehead, or chin? What about the cheeks? When trying to "type" your skin, the first thing you want to determine is how much oil you're producing. Since the Kleenex test isn't very accurate, let your eyes and a mirror tell you what you need to know.

Wash your face, then take a good look at your skin. The trick is to be objective. I think we tend to exaggerate what we see in the mirror, so try not to go overboard with your critique. It will help to give you a more accurate picture of the condition of your skin. Initially, you want to determine how clean your pores are. After washing, the superficial debris should have been rinsed away. But if you have congestion, such as blackheads, merely washing your face will not remove it. If you still see clogged pores after cleansing, you're emitting more oil than your pores can handle. The next question is where are these blackheads concentrated? Are they only on the forehead, nose, cheeks, or chin? Is the congestion concentrated in one area, or is it widespread in every pore on your face?

Oil can clog pores on your (1) forehead, (2) nose, (3) cheeks, or (4) chin. Figuring out where your pores are clogged will help you determine your skin type.

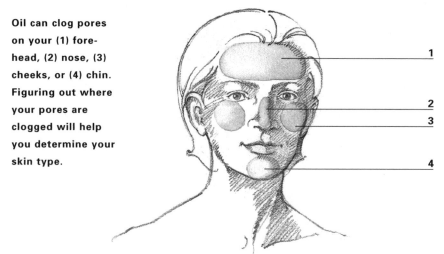

After you've summed up how much oil you're producing, there are several more questions you will want to answer. What about redness? Do you see many broken capillaries, and where are they located? Are you sensitive to almost everything you put on your skin or only certain products? Does your skin look flaky? Is it constantly peeling? Does your skin feel like it is tightly stretched over your face? How much sun exposure have you had in your lifetime? The answers to these questions will help you understand more about your skin and what to use on it.

Is your skin truly dry? I want to clear up an area of confusion regarding two very different skin types. The misunderstanding surrounds two separate conditions that are thought to be the same: dehydration and true-dry skin.

Dehydration deals with surface water loss. True-dry skin reflects a lack of oil. Many people think they have dry skin (because it *feels* dry), when really they are dehydrated. This distinction becomes very important to make when buying skin care products. If you go to the cosmetic counter and complain of dry skin—when really you are dehydrated with, let's say, normal to oily skin—you could be on the verge of a skin care catastrophe.

True-dry skin = lack of oil. Dehydrated skin = lack of water. You can be oily and dehydrated, but you cannot be both oily and dry. Your oil glands are either producing enough, too much, or not enough oil.

Although true-dry skin and dehydrated skin *feel* the same, their causes are totally different, and the treatment of each separate condition is also very different. With true-dry skin the treatment is fairly basic. The skin needs to be kept moisturized at all times. Because the sebaceous glands are not producing enough oil, you want to provide a sufficient amount of oil through product application. Exfoliation is also important to keep the dead cell buildup to a minimum. But the most important thing is to adequately hydrate true-dry skin with proper moisturizing products. Dehydration means there is an excessive dead cell buildup on the surface of your skin, and you need to exfoliate. This buildup renders your skin unable to retain water efficiently. Without regular exfoliation, the condition will continue or worsen. No amount of moisturizing will truly fix the problem, but through regular and thorough exfoliation you can greatly reduce or eliminate dehydration. Let's examine the different skin types in detail.

Dehydrated Skin

What is dehydrated skin? Dehydration is not dry skin or what I call *true-dry* skin. Dehydrated skin *feels* dry, but technically dry skin is lacking oil versus dehydrated skin that is lacking water. Dehydrated skin generally has a large buildup of dead skin cells. It is the job of those cells to retain moisture in the form of oil and water. If there are too many dead cells on the surface, more water is needed to keep all the cells moist. By eliminating the buildup (achieved through exfoliation), your cells are better able to retain moisture and less likely to become dehydrated.

Why is it dehydrated? Skin becomes dehydrated for several reasons. Some people are **genetically predisposed** and naturally dehydrated. This type of dehydration is usually very deep and tends to be harder to treat. **Climate** is a big contributor to the hydration level of the skin. People in desert climates are usually battling dehydration because there is so little moisture in the air, while those in a more humid environment don't become dehydrated as easily. **Seasonal weather** can affect the hydration of the outer skin. Winter air is usually cold and dry, coupled with indoor heat that zaps moisture from the air causing the skin to become dehydrated. Using a humidifier (see Quick Tips) to combat this dry, artificial heat can really be beneficial to the skin. **Flying** can do a number on the skin since the air in planes is extremely drying. **Sun exposure** can also leave the skin dehydrated. If, for instance, you put a bowl of water outside in the hot sun, it won't take long for the water to evaporate. The same is true for the skin. **Soap**, because it strips the skin of all oil and water, can lead to mild to severe dehydration as well.

What to use on dehydrated skin. Anytime you feel dehydrated, a good course of action would be to exfoliate, and then follow with an appropriate moisturizer. Exfoliating immediately removes dead skin buildup, enabling the remaining cells to retain water more efficiently. If you are dehydrated, yet have oily or problem skin, do not overload on moisturizer because this can easily lead to breakouts. If you're oily, using moisturizers for dry or dehydrated skin can cause clogging problems. Dehydration should be treated separately from oil or lack of oil production. In short, exfoliation is the key to alleviating dehydrated skin.

Drinking water definitely helps to keep your skin better hydrated; however, it does not eliminate dehydration. Water is utilized in your entire body for many different purposes. Even if you drink a lot of water, it doesn't necessarily go directly to your skin. But drinking at least eight 8-ounce glasses is still the rule for getting enough water in your system.

Don't use drying or harsh products on dehydrated skin. Soap can definitely cause flakiness and dehydration. Milky cleansers that are non-alkaline are best. Using an alcohol-free toner will help add moisture to the surface since most toners are primarily water. Still, the best and fastest relief for dehydrated skin is exfoliation.

True-Dry Skin

What is true-dry skin? True-dry skin is a condition where your sebaceous (oil) glands are not producing enough oil to lubricate your outer skin. The outer skin is kept moisturized by both water at the surface (and from the air) as well as sebum being excreted from your oil glands. Simply put, true-dry skin does not produce enough oil to keep the outer skin moist.

Why is it dry? The causes can be **genetic** (one or both parents had true-dry skin), or **age-related** (many people experience a slow-down in oil production as they age), or for women, **menopause**. However, many women think just because they are getting older, they will *automatically* have drier skin, but this is not necessarily the case. Sebaceous activity is not solely determined by age. A women in her late 50s may still be producing adequate amounts of oil, while a 25-year-old can have true-dry skin. **Climate** can also affect the oil glands. Dry, desert climates can cause the glands to stop or slow down oil production, just as hot climates can cause overstimulation and oilier skin.

What to use on dry skin. True-dry skin needs to be artificially lubricated with moisturizing creams. Since the oil glands are not producing enough oil to keep the skin soft, supple, and well hydrated, you want to keep high-quality moisturizers (for dry skin) on at all times. True-dry skin needs exfoliation as well since any dead cell buildup will make the skin feel even drier. The bottom line is that true-dry skin always needs a lipid or oil-based cream to make up for the lack of natural oil production.

Oily Skin

What is oily skin? This is a condition where the sebaceous glands are producing too much oil. The passageway from the oil gland to the skin's surface is via the hair follicle. Along this route, if too much oil is being produced, a traffic jam or backup will occur. This back-up produces any number of problems: blackheads (comedos or open pores), whiteheads (milia or closed pores), pustules (debris inside a closed pore is infected with pus), and potentially acne (infected cysts deep within the skin).

Why is it oily? Your skin can be oily for a number of reasons. Of course, you may be **predisposed genetically** to having oily skin. **Diet** plays a big role in how much oil is being produced. **Climate** (temperature) will affect your oil gland activity. **Heat** stimulates glandular activity, so a hot summer's day can cause your skin to be oily. **Puberty** and the onset of hormonal surges can cause oily skin to appear. Even the beginning of **menopause** can bring about fluctuations in the oil glands that can cause more oil to be produced for a period of time. **Soap**, because of its stripping action, can signal your glands to compensate by pumping out more oil. In general, your skin is oily because your sebaceous or oil glands are producing too much oil. The excess oil will just sit on the surface of your skin, making your face look and feel oily.

What to use on oily skin. Keeping oily skin clean is of the utmost importance. What you are cleansing it with is equally important. Contrary to popular opinion, you don't want to "dry out" oily skin. Drying it out *sounds* logical, but this method is ineffective and won't clear up problems. However, you do want to keep the surface cleaned out. This is done through using non-alkaline cleansers on a twice-daily basis (morning and evening). For a deep and thorough cleansing, use a clay mask once or several times per week. Finally, exfoliating actively with a gommage or scrub will help keep the dead skin buildup to a minimum. It is dead skin and oil that clog the pores, so keeping the skin clean and well exfoliated will help curb congestion.

Combination & Normal/No-Problem Skin

What is combination skin? The "t-zone," technically known as the facial axis, includes the forehead, nose, and chin area. If you have enlarged, congested pores, and/or are oily in this "t" area, you could categorize yours as combination skin.

The t-zone consists of your (1) forehead, (2) nose, and (3) chin. These areas usually contain the most active oil glands.

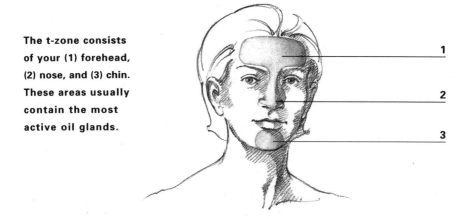

The highest concentration of active oil glands is on and around the nose. That's why almost everyone has some congestion there. The chin and forehead come next in terms of activity. Because you have more active oil glands in this t-zone region, it makes sense that you're oilier there. It is inaccurate, however, to suggest that the skin on the cheeks is dry while you have an oily t-zone. Technically, you can't have both dry and oily skin—not at the same time—so *combination*

skin is somewhat of a misnomer. Combination skin is essentially normal skin with an oily t-zone.

In comparison, normal/no-problem skin functions perfectly. It is neither too oily nor too dry. It produces enough oil without clogging the pores and maintains a high level of hydration. Normal skin rarely has any significant breakout, except perhaps during menstruation, stress, or when a poor-quality diet is involved.

Normal skin is fairly rare. Almost everyone has several things going on with his or her skin, even if there aren't any oil problems. If you have been blessed with normal/no-problem skin, you are in the minority. And, no doubt, you are the envy of the majority.

What to use. There isn't much to say about normal/no-problem skin except don't get complacent just because you don't have any problems with your skin. You can probably get away with using certain lower-quality products that may cause problems with other skin types. Even so, I recommend using high-quality products formulated for normal skin.

Not many people have no-problem skin, but those of you who do are very fortunate. You can thank your parents for the wonderful skin they have given you. However, it would be wise to exfoliate and use a clay mask regularly to help maintain your healthy, clean, and clear skin.

With combination skin, you are probably more prone to breakouts than those with normal skin. Masking, exfoliating, and using high-quality products for combination skin (normal to oily) will help keep your skin looking good and can cut down on the amount of breakout you experience. Read through the section on Oily Skin, and if you have problems with breakout, read Chapter 5 to get some ideas that can help you treat any problems you may have.

Don't get caught up using different products for different parts of your face. If you have classic combination skin, you don't need to use a cream for oily skin on your t-zone and a cream for dry skin on your cheeks. Your cheeks aren't dry (although your skin may be *dehydrated*), they just aren't overproducing oil. Products for normal to oily skin should be fine. Don't get suckered into using different creams for these different areas.

Couperose Skin

What is couperose skin? Couperose is a condition affecting the capillaries of the face. These capillaries are very thin vessels that constitute the blood network for the skin on the face. Capillaries are weak and fragile; they can "break" or dysfunction very easily. (Although the capillaries have merely dysfunctioned, many times they are termed *broken capillaries*.) When this happens, the blood stagnates within the vessels, making them more visible. Broken capillaries (couperose) look like tiny red lines under the surface of your skin. If you have thin skin, broken capillaries will be more noticeable.

Why is it couperose? This condition can happen for many different reasons. **Genetics** play a large role in how weak the capillaries are. The **environment** has a lot to do with couperose. **Sun exposure**, with its constant and **extreme heat**, can definitely cause capillary damage. Sometimes this is hard to see through a dark tan. If the tan is allowed to fade, there will usually be residual redness remaining that may be couperose. **Severely cold temperatures** or cold, windy conditions can be a cause. **Skiing** can really do a number on your skin and the capillaries. You're in cold air with the hot sun beating down while the crisp wind is hitting your face as you gracefully glide down the slopes. When skiing, your skin is vulnerable to the elements, so cover up as much as possible. It will save your skin in the long run. **Extremes in temperature** are bad for the skin and specifically the capillaries. Moderation is always best when choosing a temperature to expose your skin to. **Alcohol** and **smoking** are also culprits in causing couperose. Alcohol dilates (opens, expands) and smoking constricts (closes, contracts) the capillaries. This constant opening and/or closing can weaken the capillaries over time.

As you can see, many things contribute to couperose skin. Almost everyone by the age of 30 or 40 has a certain amount of redness to their skin—even if only in a few places. It's hard to avoid all the different factors that cause broken capillaries and still lead a normal life. People who flourish outside usually have a tough time keeping couperose away. My recommendation is to do what you can to protect your skin, then enjoy your lifestyle and activities. Life is too short.

What to use on couperose skin. In treating couperose, it's important to know what *not* to use on the skin. Capillaries are very sensitive to extremes, so you never want to use either hot or cold water directly on your face. Even going from really hot temperatures outside to cold air conditioning (and vice versa) can be hard on these vessels. Spicy foods dilate the capillaries, as do caffeine, alcohol, and sun. Smoking, air pollution, and cold or windy weather constrict the capillaries. Obviously, there are conditions that exist in our everyday lives that we cannot escape, namely the weather. Just remember to stay away from extremes whenever possible. This will help to allay further capillary damage.

Grocery and department store products rarely, if ever, address couperose skin, but many professional product lines do. Keep in mind, nothing will get rid of existing broken capillaries, so *prevention* should be the focus. Avoid extremes and use products specifically formulated to tone or promote proper capillary function.

Sensitive Skin

What is sensitive skin? There are two different kinds of sensitive skin. There is the kind that is sensitive to the touch and the kind that *feels* sensitive. If you have the kind that is sensitive to the touch, it just means your skin tends to turn red merely by being touched. I have several clients who turn bright red merely by lightly touching their faces. This type of sensitive skin is of little concern when figuring out your skin type. Reactive skin or skin that *feels* sensitive will itch, burn, or feel irritated when certain disagreeable products are applied. There are many ingredients in the world of cosmetics that can irritate even nonsensitive skin, let alone someone with sensitivities.

You usually know if you have sensitive skin. You've experienced it firsthand over the years. You've tried dozens of products and skin care lines and have probably reacted to many. If you've finally discovered something that doesn't cause a reaction, you'll be prone to sticking with what you've found for fear of getting "burned"—literally.

It's hard to determine exactly what products and which ingredients are causing your skin to turn red, burn, or breakout. In case you haven't discovered the ill effects of the following ingredient on your own, let me advise you: stay away from products that contain *fragrance*. Many companies add fragrance to their products. A lot of the department store product lines started out as perfumeries and then branched out into skin care and cosmetics. They tend to add their signature fragrance to all (or most) of the products in their line, distinguishing them at least aromatically as their own. These products may smell good, but if you have sensitive skin, watch out. Perfumes and fragrances are *not* good (or desirable) ingredients for skin care products. If you are sensitive, your skin will no doubt let you know. Along with skin sensitivities, many people are simply allergic to fragrance. (See Chapter 15/Fragrances of Old.)

Why is it sensitive? Sensitivities can be caused for many reasons. You may have **inherited** sensitive skin from one or both parents. You may have spent a lifetime using **harsh soaps** and **drying products** on your skin that will inevitably lead to sensitivities. If you have or are currently using **Retin-A**, or have had strong glycolic or chemical **peels**, your skin will no doubt be sensitive. **Laser resurfacing** may also bring about long-term sensitivities. **Couperose** skin tends to be sensitive because the capillaries sit so close to the surface and can be reactive. **Thin skin** is usually more sensitive than thick skin. Thin skin is less impervious to irritants than thick, more protective skin. And finally, skin that has been abused in the **sun** can become sensitive over time.

What to use on sensitive skin. It may be easier to list what *not* to use on sensitive skin since what you can use will vary greatly depending on how sensitive you are. You want to avoid abrasive scrubs. Although exfoliation is vital to healthy skin, you don't want to cause more sensitivity by using a harsh scrub. Just imagine rubbing abrasive particles on sensitive skin. It doesn't even sound good, and it will feel even worse. Soap is another undesirable product. People with sensitive skin want to be especially careful to use only non-alkaline products on their skin. This is very important. Once again, avoid fragrance as an ingredient in your face products. Fragrance will almost always cause a reaction even on skins that aren't considered sensitive. Heat will further exacerbate sensitive skin. As with burns, you want to treat the skin gently, never using anything extreme. You must avoid strong peels. These will do little to benefit the skin and can go a long way to furthering any sensitivities and redness you may already have. It is doubtful a person with very sensitive skin would be able to tolerate a strong peel, but high-percentage acid peels should definitely be avoided. The sun and wind can cause irritation with any skin, especially sensitive skin. Try to cover up as much of your face as possible in cold and/or sunny conditions.

Recommending what to use on sensitive skin will vary based on the oil content of your skin and the origin of the sensitivities. Most product lines address sensitivities, but a sensitive skin type will probably go through more trial and error using products than other kinds of skin.

Sun-Damaged Skin

What is sun-damaged skin? Sun-damaged skin isn't so much a skin type as it is the outcome of long-term overexposure to the sun. This sort of skin usually comes on a type of person—the outdoors type. Sun-damaged skin is characterized by rough, dried-out skin with a lot of deep wrinkles. The epidermis or outer skin tends to be thickened (a natural, protective response to sun exposure), and there is usually significant loss of elasticity or "firmness" to the skin. Your skin becomes what is technically termed *flaccid*. Deep, often premature wrinkles are present along with noticeable capillary damage. Many times sun-damaged skin has a leathered look and almost always is sporting a continuous tan.

Sometimes sun-damaged skin isn't currently tan. Although excessive sun exposure may have stopped, prematurely wrinkled and flaccid skin may have already occurred from damage acquired years ago. This is what cumulative, long-term damage can mean. Long after you have stayed out of the sun, the effects of overexposure still creep into your life, showing up not *only* in the form of lines, wrinkles, and loose skin, but also with the potential for skin cancer or precancerous growths as well.

Why is it sun damaged? The one and only explanation for sun-damaged skin is—**sun**. Continual, long-term exposure is what causes sun-damaged skin.

What to use on sun-damaged skin. You want to treat the oil or lack of oil in your skin first and foremost. If you have truly sun-damaged skin, there isn't anything—short of invasive procedures—to reduce or eliminate the damage. Is your skin oily? Couperose? Sensitive? Deciding what other skin conditions you have, coupled with sun damage, will be the determining factors for what is best to use on your skin.

There are no quick fixes for a lifetime spent in the sun. You can help to stop further damage by avoiding direct sunlight and always wearing sunscreen and a hat. Read through Chapter 10 for detailed information about the sun and sun protection. Just remember, it's never too late to start taking care of your skin—no matter what condition it is in.

Mature Skin

Mature skin is commonly used to describe a skin type, but actually, the word *mature* is arbitrary and only suggests the person in question is older. But how old? Old enough to have true-dry skin? Yes, as you age the oil glands tend to put out less and less oil, but even someone in her 20s can have true-dry skin. Would she use a cream for mature skin? Products for mature skin usually have special ingredients that repair and regenerate skin that has "broken down." But many people could use these special benefits even though their skin may not be classified "mature."

My issue with mature skin products is the marketing approach: trying to get older people to buy special (usually more expensive) creams. These products may manipulate older people into thinking they can repair a lifetime of natural aging when actually they cannot undo the past. My contention is that everybody—every skin—has specific and special regeneration needs, not just mature skin.

Finally, if a person with mature skin doesn't actually have dry skin and uses one of these specialized products with a lot of oils in a heavy cream, watch out! As I've stated before, age and true-dry skin don't necessarily go hand in hand. You are not guaranteed to have oil-deficient skin as you get older. It's just not as simple as that. If you go to the department store and someone sells you a mature skin moisturizer, unless you do have true-dry skin, you could be headed for some skin care problems, most likely congestion or clogged pores.

Be careful how you classify your skin. Skin type should start with how much (or how little) oil your skin is producing. This is based on you as an individual, not on your age.

Quick Tips

- Humidifiers add moisture to the air. If you have dehydrated skin, I recommend putting a humidifier in your bedroom and using it nightly—especially in winter. Your skin will be a "captive audience" for the six to eight hours you are asleep. It can make a big difference in the moisture level of your skin. Remember to keep the humidifier away from direct contact with your furniture. (It can warp the wood due to all the moisture.)

- Whenever you have a facial, be sure to ask the aesthetician, "What's my skin type?" Hopefully you will get the same answer from any professional you go to. This information will help you when purchasing products on your own.

Problem Skin

From the occasional breakout to full-blown acne, hardly anyone escapes problems with his or her skin from time to time.
Although the causes are many, I believe you can keep breakouts to a minimum when armed with knowledge and a bit of
common sense. Since the different manifestations of problem
skin stem from similar causes, I recommend reading this entire
chapter. You may pick up helpful information in a section you
didn't think pertained to you. Some recommendations overlap
and are listed in Problem Solvers at the end of this chapter.
Let's take a look at some of the major skin care problems and
their possible solutions.

Breakout

What is breakout? Breakout is like a traffic jam inside your hair follicle or pore. The follicle is like a passageway or tunnel. Oil (sebum) comes up through the follicle and out onto the surface of your skin, picking up dead cells along the way. When too much oil tries to get through at any given time, and/or there are too many dead cells sticking to the follicle wall, it starts a chain reaction resulting in a backup. For instance, when traffic starts to slow down on the highway (follicle), it causes a traffic jam (congestion) with an eventual backup (breakout) that can go on for miles.

Once this backup has started, the amount of oil within the follicle starts to increase. This buildup causes the follicle wall to expand and eventually break. Bacteria rush in, which in turn increases the infection. Now you have a hard, red, and sometimes large bump under your skin, commonly referred to as a pimple, zit, or blemish. Technically it is a pustule (if it has a white or yellow pus-filled head), or a cyst or papule (a bump lurking under the skin that contains infection but has no visible head).

Why does skin break out? Quite simply, hormones cause breakouts. Hormones are little chemical messengers that tell your glands what to do. In the case of your skin, hormones control the oil or sebaceous glands. *Why* the hormones are being activated is what we want to know. The major factors that contribute to breakouts are hormone imbalance, diet, stress, and genetics.

Hormonal imbalances can occur at any time in life. As **puberty** starts, the hormones are activated. This is the first real opportunity for any significant breakout to occur. For women, because of our **monthly cycles**, breakouts can happen as frequently as once a month throughout our childbearing years. Any irregularities with the monthly cycle can lead to skin problems as well. **Pregnancy** causes great hormonal changes and can either improve your complexion or cause mild to severe breakout. Finally comes **menopause**, bringing yet another change in a woman's hormone levels. It is not unusual for a **perimenopausal** (the precursor to menopause) woman to experience some breakout. The hormones are fluctuating, and even at this stage of your life, you can still be plagued with blemishes.

Many people believe it is during puberty that breakout should occur and not any time afterwards. Countless clients come to my office in disbelief that they are 30, 40, or even 50 years old, yet they're still experiencing breakout. Puberty is usually the first time breakout makes an appearance, but due to all the previously mentioned hormonal fluctuations in a woman's life, breakout can occur at any time, no matter what your age. And although men don't have a monthly menstrual cycle, bear children, or go through menopause, their hormones are in flux at different stages of their lives as well.

Diet is a huge consideration when looking for the cause(s) of breakout. I have read many books and heard many dermatologists say food doesn't affect the skin, cause breakouts, or exacerbate acne. I wholeheartedly disagree! I believe food can affect your mood, your energy level, your general health, and of course your skin. To say that a diet laden with **sugary, fatty, deep-fried,** or **fast food** doesn't have a negative effect on the skin makes no sense. In my professional experience, it is rare for a client to come in with breakout and not also have a poor diet. Yes, someone may eat a well-balanced diet and also have a hormone imbalance that is causing major eruptions. But nine times out of ten, a person with breakout is also a person who could use some dietary changes for the better.

Stress should not be overlooked as being a factor in skin troubles. Stress can come in many forms but always puts a strain on the body as a whole. Even short-term stressors can cause a breakdown in the body's immune system, weakening its defense against invaders. Clients come to me all the time with breakout caused by **short-**

and **long-term stresses** they are experiencing in their lives. Stress is very hard on the body overall, which in turn puts a strain on the organs of elimination such as the liver, kidneys, colon, and skin. Taking care to eat well during periods of stress is extremely important, as well as considering taking vitamin and mineral supplements to help your body out in its time of need.

Did one or both of your parents have acne or problem skin as teenagers? Did they have problems at any other time in their lives? If the answer is "yes" to either of these questions, you may be **predisposed genetically** to problem skin at some point in your life. And if you or your spouse had hormonally charged skin as a teenager or even later in life, you may have passed that down to your kids. Even someone with the cleanest diet, living a healthy lifestyle, may not escape an inherited trait for problem skin.

There are many reasons for breakout, and they usually involve a mixture of the previously mentioned causes in varying degrees. Unlike people with normal, no-problem skin, those of you with problems will have to dedicate a bit more time and energy to keep your breakouts to a minimum. Clear skin might not come easily, but I'm quite sure it is within your reach. Willingness to change, commitment to a program, understanding why you're broken out, and patience with your body's healing process will help get you there.

Pressure breakout. Sometimes continually sleeping on one side of your face will cause a kind of pressure breakout. Football helmets, chin straps, and sweatbands are a few more possible causes of pressure-induced skin problems. This type of sports gear can inhibit elimination, causing sweat to pile up in certain areas, which can cause irritation and potential breakout.

Sometimes a client will come in with a significant amount of breakout on only one side of her face. If it is predominately around the left or right chin area, I ask which side of her face she holds the phone up to.

Usually it's the same side where the breakout has occurred. Telephones get dirty quickly and easily, and we tend to rest the phone on our faces unconsciously. The buildup of oil and makeup can be transferred to the skin and cause irritation and possibly small breakouts. When using public or pay phones, just imagine how many people have used the same telephone. If it's bad to let your own phone rest on your face, you really don't want a pay phone touching your skin. There is no telling what is on the end of that receiver!

What to do for breakouts. There are several beneficial things you can do for existing breakouts that will help them to go away without causing any damage to your skin. Please keep in mind, once a blemish has made its presence known, nothing is going to get rid of it overnight. Usually, the more you try to conceal the problem, the more noticeable you make it. Being gentle works better than being unkind to the skin. Patience and allowing time to take care of the healing process along with understanding why you're having the breakout in the first place will help in the long run.

The red look of a blemish indicates there is infection present. Infection creates inflammation (thus the red color). If something is inflamed, it is holding heat, and the last thing you want to put on an infected area is more heat (for example, hot compresses). It would be like running hot water over a finger you just burned on the stove. These spots need to be soothed, not irritated further.

Applying benzoyl peroxide and other drying agents will also irritate the skin. These "zit zappers" contain harsh ingredients meant to dry out the blemish. What they really do is dry up the water in the surrounding tissue, which causes the skin to dry and flake. It may *seem* like you've solved the problem, but the infection just sits there—dormant—waiting for another chance to flare up. You've also irritated the surrounding tissue and caused it to flake, prolonging the healing process.

The following recommendations are not miracle cures, but are far superior to any spot or acne treatments available on the market. For common small to medium breakout, these next two products can go a long way in helping your skin look its best.

A clay mask is my number one at-home treatment for breakout. As discussed in Chapter 2, clay is a natural healer. It has a calming effect and helps to temporarily lift redness from the skin. Clay draws to itself, helping to encourage movement of the debris in an imbedded pore. It is antiseptic, which helps to keep bacteria away. The mask also acts as an occlusive cover to shield the blemish from the outside air while the clay's healing powers go to work.

Clay can be used in two ways: as a mask, covering the entire face and left on for 15 minutes once or twice a week, or dotted on the blemishes at night before bed and left on while you sleep. (If you are going to be home for an extended period of time, you can dot the clay on during the day if that works better for you. Leave it on as long as you can, at least 30 minutes.) If the spot is small to medium without a lot of infection, this dotting method can really reduce its size overnight. For deeper cysts and large infected areas, clay can still do wonders, but not miracles.

Essential oil of geranium is my next wonder treatment for breakout. After you have completed your Basic 1-2-3 routine, dot geranium oil directly on any infected (red) blemishes. Essential oils are discussed in Chapter 8, but I will list just a few of their attributes here. Please note: DO NOT get geranium or *any* pure essential oil in or around your eyes!

Essential oils are not "oily" oils; they are more gaseous and vaporous. They have a thin viscosity and do not feel oily. By their very nature, essential oils are antiseptic, antibacterial, and in many cases soothing, which makes them perfect for infections. Unlike having clay dots on your face, you can dab essential oils on your spots, and aside from the natural aromatics, no one will be the wiser.

Essential oil of geranium is especially good for problem skin. It has antiseptic and astringent properties as well as a balancing action on oil production. Geranium also helps to stop bleeding and promote healing of injured areas.

You want to purchase *pure* essential oils. They are usually easy to find in larger health food stores. Because pure essential oils cannot be housed in plastic, make sure the oils you purchase are in glass bottles. Essential oils are heat-sensitive. Left in a hot environment or exposed to sunlight, all of the active properties in the bottle of oil will be destroyed. Thus they are commonly found in dark blue or brown glass bottles. Usually they come in an easy to use 1/3- to 1/2-ounce bottle with a dropper top. This size ought to last you for months. A very small amount will go a long way.

Some of my clients don't like geranium's aroma. Because pure essential oils are undiluted, their aromatics are quite potent. You will usually know immediately if you like a particular smell or not. If geranium is not to your liking, essential oil of juniper is a good alternative. Juniper is antiseptic, purifying, and has detoxifying actions. Essential oil of lavender is usually well tolerated by most people's noses. French lavender (sometimes called lavender "fine") is most commonly used. Lavender is antiseptic, antibacterial, and is also soothing to the nerves. Although juniper and lavender are good alternatives, the best essential oil for your blemishes is geranium.

Combining a clay mask with geranium oil is the most effective overnight treatment for blemishes. After you've completed your evening 1-2-3 program, dot some clay mask on any problem spots and let it dry for a minute or so. Then take your geranium oil and dab a bit on top of the clay and leave it overnight. In the morning you should see some reduction in size along with diminished redness of the blemish. Continue this dotting method for several consecutive nights or until the blemish is gone.

Breakout is one instance when essential oils and clay are ideal. Even though you may have to contend with red spots already present on your face, these products will go a long way to help expedite the healing process. There is no fast and easy way to get rid of blemishes. They weren't created instantaneously, and they will not disappear overnight. Give a clay mask and essential oils a try, and see if they don't work better for your skin than the blemish-control products you've been using.

Keep in mind that problems with your skin are internal. Treating them topically will help, but it will not keep the blemishes from appearing. You have to understand this in order to take hold of the problem. If you continue to treat them from the outside, you are only treating the symptom (breakout), and you are fighting a losing battle. You must also go after the cause (hormones, diet, stress). This course of action will take longer and tends to seem harder because it doesn't merely involve applying an ointment or taking a pill. Causal healing requires commitment, and in some cases abstinence, as well as a true desire to change. When things aren't working (you're still breaking out), it's time for a change.

Extractions. I *do not* recommend extracting your own skin. This is one skill better left to a professional. Since I know it's futile to think you won't pick at your skin (I have many clients who are addicted), I am including the following guidelines for you to follow. Please know this: your zit has a mind of its own, and it will *always win*. You're trying to make something *less* noticeable, but after self-extracting you usually end up with the opposite effect. By using the following rules it is my hope that you will at least not scar or damage your skin.

Rule #1: Always wrap your fingers in tissue. I want to emphasize the importance of this simple step. Even if you just washed your hands, you still want to protect against bacteria, not to mention your fingernails. Take a tissue, fold it in half, then tear it in half, and use the two folded halves to wrap around your index fingers.

Rule #2: There must be a *clear* and *defined* head on the blemish, or it is *not* extractable. Many blemishes are actually cysts underneath the surface that *cannot be extracted*. In trying to remove debris from one of these cyst-type spots, you will drive the infection further down into the skin, forcing it into the surrounding tissue. This will cause the blemish to get bigger, look redder, and take longer to go away. Scarring is a possible result from trying to extract these unextractable places.

Rule #3: After one or two tries, leave it alone. If you've tried to extract a certain spot and after a few attempts the debris won't budge, *leave it alone*. I think this is the hardest rule to follow. It requires self-discipline and control, something a lot of self-extractors don't have too much of. If you continue to pick at a place relentlessly, you will most likely scar your skin. There is no way around this. Debris comes out when it's ready. Pressing harder or going at it longer won't change this fact; it will only cause harm to your skin.

Comedos (common blackheads) by definition are open pores. Usually they will extract without giving you trouble. Still, if the debris doesn't want to come out, follow Rule #3 and leave it alone.

Rule #4: You must treat the places you've extracted. At the very least, put a dot of a clay mask on any spots you've just picked at. This will help soothe the area and help fight bacterial infection. Please don't leave these places as open, untreated wounds and just walk away. If you're going to pick, you must do it correctly. If you can, leave the clay on for at least 5-10 minutes. Essential oil of geranium is antibacterial and can be applied directly to the spots as well.

Here is what I *really* recommend. As your fingers are approaching your face, warming up to do a fantastic picking job, change their direction and grab your clay mask instead. Put it on the spots and walk away from the mirror. You have just put something beneficial on your blemishes while not incurring any damage through picking. Congratulations! This is always the best course of action to follow. If your skin is in need of extractions, I recommend getting a facial and letting a professional do this delicate work.

Blackheads & Whiteheads

What is a blackhead? Technically termed a *comedo* or *comedone*, a blackhead is an open pore clogged with debris (dead skin and oil or sebum). A comedone is dark or black because oil inside the pore reacts to the oxygen in the air (it oxidizes) and turns dark. Tiny specks of melanin (the dark pigment in your skin) are also present in blackheads, contributing to their color. Blackheads are considered noninflammatory and contain no infection.

Why do blackheads occur? As described earlier, blackheads form as a result of too much oil trying to get to the surface. The pore can only handle so much oil at one time. The result is congestion (clogging) and a blackhead or plug is formed. The reason for this excess oil can be **hormonal, dietary,** or **genetic.** Sometimes using a **cream** (moisturizer) that is too heavy can cause clogging. Alkaline **soaps** strip the skin of oil and water, sometimes making the oil glands pump more oil to compensate for the loss. This can create blackheads.

What to do for blackheads. Keeping the skin clean through daily cleansing is the first step for reducing the potential for blackheads. Since dead skin and oil clog the pores, getting rid of this surface debris will help maintain cleaner skin. Exfoliation is another important step in keeping blackheads away. Regular exfoliation keeps the surface of your skin smooth and free from a buildup of accumulated dead cells. This, therefore, helps to keep the pores from clogging. Finally, using a clay mask will deep clean open pores, helping to keep blackheads to a minimum.

What is a whitehead? Whiteheads (also termed *milia*) are closed pores that are clogged. They contain the same debris as blackheads, but since there is no pore opening, the debris in a whitehead has nowhere to go. Because dead skin covers the opening to the pore, sebum doesn't mix with oxygen in the air and therefore maintains its natural white or yellowish color. Thus the term *whitehead*. Milia are also considered to be noninflammatory.

Why do whiteheads occur? Whiteheads can form for similar reasons as blackheads: **hormones, genetics,** and **heavy creams**. I have found clients who consume large amounts of **dairy products** (mainly milk) tend to form a lot of whiteheads. The forehead seems to be the primary place for these dairy-induced milia to show up. **Dehydration** can sometimes cause whiteheads. When the dead cell buildup is thick, layers of dead skin easily cover the pores, creating milia.

What to do for whiteheads. Since whiteheads by definition are closed pores, an opening must be made in order for the debris to come out. Therefore, I recommend having milia professionally removed. I am not a proponent of self-extracting, especially in the case of milia or any other closed pores. In the case of whiteheads, self-extraction can lead to disaster. Trying to extract whiteheads without creating an opening will force the debris farther down into the follicle wall, causing the potential for infection and a much more noticeable problem.

Usually a whitehead continues to grow, like a snowball rolling down a mountain, continuing to collect debris that has nowhere to escape. Large milia are easier for an aesthetician to extract.

The debris will be forced to the surface due to its ever-increasing size, and through professional extraction it can be removed for good.

The simple rule to follow for self-extracting is this: blackheads (open pores) are usually extractable, whiteheads (because they are closed pores) are not.

Teen Skin

Many of my clients have asked what they can do for their teenagers' problem skin. Or sometimes they simply want to start their teens on a good skin care program, but don't know where to begin. Whether your kids have problem skin or not, there are some basic habits teenagers should try to develop that can have a positive effect on their skin. I have written this section especially for them.

1. Keeping your skin clean is of paramount importance. Generally, you use soap to wash your face. This presents problem number one. Almost all soaps have high alkalinity. Alkaline cleansers should not be used, especially by people (young or old) having problems with their skin.

To refresh your memory, alkalinity strips all surface oil and water off your skin, leaving it depleted. The oil glands will usually pump out more oil to compensate for the loss. Adding to this excess oil, your skin might become dehydrated from the soap. So your face may *feel* dry (although it's simple dehydration), yet will look and feel oily at the same time. Confusing, isn't it? Liquid Aveeno or Cetaphil (cleansers mentioned in Chapter 1) would be good alternatives to soap. They are inexpensive and do a good job of cleansing.

So keeping the skin clean with a non-alkaline cleanser is the first rule to follow. Just as I would instruct adults, you should be washing your face both in the morning and in the evening. Getting into good skin care habits early on will benefit you down the road.

2. Rinse off your face immediately after exercising. This is very important. All that salty sweat is basically toxic waste (toxins) being released from your body. It is coming out of your body, and you need to complete the elimination by thoroughly rinsing your face with water until you can't taste the saltiness anymore. Many clients who were experiencing sweat-related problems had a significant reduction in their breakouts using this quick rinse-off method.

3. Don't wash too much. If clean is good, then surely washing several times throughout the day must be better, right? Well, it's not. Since soap dries out the surface of your skin, you are essentially forcing your oil glands to pump and pump and pump to keep the surface lubricated. Even using non-alkaline cleansers can overstimulate the oil glands, giving rise to oilier skin. Although it is important to keep the skin clean, you don't want to create more oil. Washing twice a day is a good guideline—and always after sweating. If you feel the need to wash another time in the day, then do so. But in general, don't wash too much.

4. Abrasive scrubs are *out* if there are problems with infection (red bumps, pimples, blemishes, zits, and/or acne). Blemishes can easily be opened up or irritated with the abrasive particles contained in a scrub. Like open wounds, a scrub can leave these blemishes subject to even more infection and make them take longer to heal. If no infection is present, scrubs are fine to use—as long as they are used with care. You never want to rub too aggressively with a scrub.

5. Pimple-drying agents should not be used on problem skin. This includes benzoyl peroxide, blemish pads, etc. These products are very harsh, to say the least. They're being used on skin that is infected and inflamed. This tissue needs soothing, calming, antibacterial products used on it, not harsh, caustic creams. For information on useful products, see the section "What to do for breakouts" earlier in this chapter.

6. Food *does* affect your skin. As I've said previously, there are plenty of books and many doctors who will disagree with me on this issue. However, I have seen too much evidence to believe otherwise. It just doesn't make sense that what you eat doesn't affect everything about you, including your skin. It's like saying I can fill up my car's gas tank with orange juice, and this won't affect how it runs. A car requires a certain type of fuel to run efficiently, and so does your body. If you put low-quality foods into your system, sooner or later your system (your body) will rebel.

When someone comes to see me with breakout, the first questions I ask concern their diet (daily intake of food). This includes questions about sugar intake as well. I have found over and over that poor diet and excess consumption of sugar (along with other factors) equals skin trouble. This is not to say someone with problem skin couldn't be eating well but have a hormone imbalance that is causing problems. I've seen that too. But more often than not, diet plays a key role in how clear (or broken out) your skin is.

During the teen years (I know this was true for me), eating healthy, well-balanced meals isn't necessarily the norm. There tends to be a lot of sodas and sweets, and usually a more than occasional fast-food burger and fries. Even if your stomach can survive this, it is doubtful your skin will—not for any extended length of time. I think your body can tolerate all kinds of abuse for a short period of time, but after your time is up, your body will rebel. It will start creating symptoms of overload. One of these "symptoms" is breakout.

And to top that off, kids are bombarded by advertisements to use spot treatment this or zit remover that. As I've said before, these products do little more than irritate the skin and put the eruption in a dormant (inactive, not cleared up) state. Become aware of how food may be affecting your skin.

7. Don't pick. I know this is an impossible request. I feel it is my duty to at least address this issue even though I'm quite sure faces will be picked at by their owners. It's human nature. Earlier in this chapter was a list of rules to follow if you can't stay away from your face. But truly, my recommendation is to leave your face alone. Use the treatments described in the Breakout section, but otherwise don't pick at your face.

When to start your kids on a skin care program. When your children are starting puberty, it would be beneficial to start them on a good skin care program. If they aren't having any problems with their skin, at least make sure they are cleansing morning and night with a non-alkaline cleanser. That's a good start, and later down the road you can add other products (toners and moisturizers, exfoliators and masks) when needed. But at such a young age, and if no problems are present, their skin is functioning optimally and won't need a lot of extra care.

If your teens are having problems, it's time to get them started on a good program of cleansing, exfoliating, and using a clay mask to help keep their breakouts to a minimum. Discussed in detail in Chapter 2, exfoliating and using a clay mask are additional steps that can help make a difference in their skin.

Numerous clients have found good results for their teenagers' skin by following the previously mentioned steps in this section (and throughout this chapter). Not all teenagers are going to follow a skin care routine, but I have found that if they see good results from following a simple program, they will be more prone to follow through with it on a regular basis.

Acne

Acne is something you wouldn't wish on anybody. Yet many of us will have to contend with it sometime in our lives. It can be debilitating and embarrassing and can cause real psychological scars that stay with us for a long time. Unfortunately, the scars can be physical as well. In this section, I am not proposing a cure or some miracle program to stop acne from occurring, but I will explain what it is and provide some suggestions for coping with this disease. As a teenager, I had (what I remember to be) perfect skin. It wasn't until I was 23 that I developed a case of acne that I will never forget. It doesn't matter when it hits you, it is devastating. So I hope you never have to go through what we acne sufferers have gone through. And if you have acne now (or know someone who does), hopefully there will be some information here that you find helpful, which can lead you to a path of healthier skin—for a lifetime.

What is acne? The following has been reprinted with permission from Johnson & Johnson, Inc. They so clearly explain how acne develops, I wanted to pass the information along to you as it was written.

Long before blemishes appear on your skin, trouble has been building up beneath the surface— in the hair follicles and their attached oil glands.

As you can see in Figure 1, each follicle contains a number of sebaceous or oil glands. The oil you see on your skin is sebum, which comes from these glands.

Cells that line the follicle surrounding the hair are being constantly replaced. They mix with sebum and work their way to the surface of the skin. Eventually they are washed away. Sometimes,

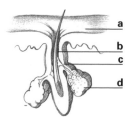

Figure 1:
Normal hair follicle
a) skin surface
b) cells
c) sebum
d) sebaceous glands

however, this process goes haywire. For reasons not completely understood, the follicle begins to produce cells that stick together so tightly that they are not shed. Accumulated cells, bound up in sebum and mixed with other skin materials, including pigment and bacteria, stick together and form a plug. This plug clogs up the pore, obstructing the opening to the skin. But the sebaceous gland keeps producing sebum, and this is how acne begins. The initial buildup is called a microcomedo (Figure 2). It lies deep within the follicle and starts forming many weeks before you notice any disturbance on your skin.

The sebaceous gland continues to put oil into the blocked system, and the follicle begins to swell and forms a closed comedo or whitehead (Figure 3). A whitehead is usually visible as a slight bump on the skin. If the follicle doesn't break, the whitehead may turn into an open comedo or blackhead (Figure 4). The familiar blackhead is like a whitehead except that the exit to the skin surface is open. Some of the materials in the follicle cause it to darken. This material, and not dirt, gives the blackhead its dark color. Often the follicle bursts or leaks from the pressure in the plugged system. A papule or pimple (Figure 5) forms when the follicle begins to release its contents into the surrounding tissue, causing inflammation. That's why the skin surface surrounding a pimple usually appears reddened and swollen.

The white cells in the body attack this material and pus develops. These pus-filled inflammations are called pustules (Figure 6) and in about 10 days

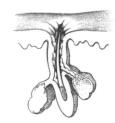

Figure 2: Microcomedo

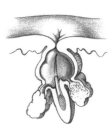

Figure 3: Whitehead or closed comedo

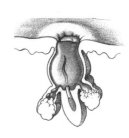

Figure 4: Blackhead or open comedo

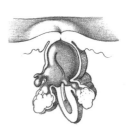

Figure 5: Papule

will usually disappear by themselves as the body disposes of this material.

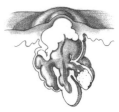

You might suffer from whiteheads, blackheads, papules or pustules or a combination of all of them. Keep in mind that these blemishes are just expressions of acne at different stages of development. But every one originated from a microcomedo hidden within the follicle—which is why we say acne is a problem that works against you from the inside out.

What to use on acne skin. In order to really treat acne, I truly believe you must get your entire house in order. Don't just look for topical or oral medications from your dermatologist to work miracles on your skin. It really takes a commitment to proper eating habits, a good skin care program, staying away from picking at the skin, and sometimes using prescription topical or oral medications to further reduce the lesions on your face.

If you have acne, products and facials—although helpful— are not the sole answer. I believe you must also look to your diet. Please don't discount the possibility that what you are putting in your mouth is having an effect on your skin. I highly recommend getting in touch with a clinical nutritionist or someone who really understands the relationship between food and skin. I believe you have to go to the source of the problem (in this case, food being a potential contributing factor) rather than merely treating the symptom, which is problem skin. Hormones are the primary cause of skin problems, but food does have a secondary effect.

For those of you with acne, I recommend following the Basic 1-2-3 program (cleansing, toning, and hydrating with a moisturizer specifically made for problem skin), along with diligent exfoliating with a gel peel or gommage, plus a clay mask. Whenever there are problems with the skin, exfoliating and masking should be done at least two or three times per week. Read Chapter 2 (The Extras) along with this whole chapter to get more ideas on what to use on your skin.

Acne is an exterior sign of internal imbalance. Look at your diet, hormone fluctuations, and how you are taking care of your skin. All of these have to be in balance in order to control and eventually clear acne.

Adult acne. I have many clients who have been diagnosed as having adult acne. Upon further examination, it turns out they simply have a minor breakout. Usually it is caused by improper diet, stress, or perhaps a hormone imbalance. I dislike the term *adult acne*, although it is widely used nowadays to describe problem skin in adults. Technically, even a blackhead has the potential for acne. But it is rare in these individuals diagnosed with adult acne that I see true acne, as opposed to a small breakout. It is all a matter of degree, but the kind of acne I use the term *acne* for is the full-blown type. I don't like over-using the term *adult acne* because it makes a minor breakout sound much more intense than it really is, lessening the weight of having true acne.

Problem Solvers

In order to gain control of problem skin, there are a few important items that should not be overlooked. Although I have already mentioned some of the following problem solvers, I am repeating them here as a consolidated body of information you can easily refer to. If you can incorporate all of these into your day, although there are no guarantees, I would be surprised if you did not see some marked improvement in your skin. These are not in any particular order of importance, but they are all important for keeping your body—and therefore your skin—healthy, inside and out.

Water. Drinking enough water throughout the day will really help your body get rid of toxins. Water is in no way a cure-all, but without it all of your eliminating organs (including your skin) have to work harder. The goal is to make it *easier* for your body to eliminate toxins. Eight 8-ounce glasses a day is the minimum to maintain healthy cells and overall hydration. I don't recommend tap water because it contains chemicals, such as chlorine. Purchase clean, filtered water or get a water filter for your tap.

No sugar (of any kind). If you follow this one piece of advice, it will go a long way to helping your skin clear up. I have seen this to be true in my own skin as well as dozens of my clients throughout the years. Sugar is a major contributor to problem skin. (See Chapter 13/Sugar.)

Chlorophyll. For anyone experiencing breakout, I recommend reading about chlorophyll in Chapter 14. In short, chlorophyll acts as an internal cleanser, helping to eliminate toxins from the body. It's a health aid in numerous ways, but I have had a lot of clients find good results by taking "nature's green drink" to help with their problem skin.

Evening primrose oil can help to reduce the amount of oil produced by the sebaceous glands. In some cases it can help to reduce breakouts. (See Chapter 14/Evening Primrose Oil.)

No sun exposure if you can help it. I'm not saying don't go outside; I mean no *direct* sunlight on your face. Heat activates all glandular activity, including your oil glands. Sometimes you can't help getting exposure, but certainly don't purposefully bask in the sun thinking it will clear up your problem skin. It won't. In fact, with the worst case scenario, it will increase the amount of breakout you are experiencing. If you have to be in the sun, wear protection such as a wide-brimmed hat, and as always, wear sunscreen. (See Chapter 16/Myth: Sun clears up acne.)

Don't wash too much. This has the potential to stimulate the sebaceous glands and create more oil. Twice a day and anytime after you have been sweating is all you need. Don't think cleaning the surface will eliminate the problem. Try to look at the problems with your skin as stemming from an imbalance on the inside, not just breakout on the outside. And remember, no soaps; only use non-alkaline cleansers.

Don't let sweat dry on your skin. Immediately rinse your face with water after exercising. You don't ever want sweat to dry on the surface of your skin. Otherwise you're just asking for trouble.

Break it down. Try to break down the different elements in your life to find possible causes for your breakouts. If it's a new breakout, what is new in your life? Are you using new skin care products, shampoo, even laundry detergent? Have you eaten new or unusual foods you don't normally eat? Have you eaten more sugar than you ordinarily eat? Is it Halloween or your birthday? Have the Girl Scouts been coming around? Has your monthly cycle changed? Are you going through puberty? What about the amount of stress in your life? Try to break down your lifestyle habits to see if there is a correlation between something you're doing, eating, or not doing, and how this may be affecting your skin. Breakout usually has multiple causes, but eliminating the ones you think might be contributing to your skin problems is a good start to clearer skin.

There are no guarantees that any of the suggestions in this chapter will completely or even partially clear up your problem skin. I offer them because in my experience with my clients, they have had good results incorporating some or all of these recommendations. There are many routes to healthy, clear skin. The road I prefer is getting to the cause of the problem and trying to fix it from the inside out.

If your skin gets beyond your control, and you don't feel comfortable altering your diet and lifestyle habits, perhaps you would be a good candidate for seeking out a dermatologist's care. He or she will be able to prescribe oral and/or topical medications that have been proven to help people with problem skin. My feeling, however, is that whichever route you choose, if you don't alter your diet and eliminate poor-quality foods such as sugar, you are doing your skin a huge disservice.

Problem skin begs for attention. And although it takes commitment, perseverance, and patience, I know you can experience trouble-free skin if you are willing to be open to change. In life, I believe anything is possible.

Checklist for Problem Skin

Do:

Be diligent with your Basic 1-2-3 program

Make sure you include The Extras 1-3 times per week

Eat well (lots of fruits & vegetables)

Drink a lot of water

Try chlorophyll, 4 tablespoons in water 2 times a day (See page 205)

Try evening primrose oil (See page 211)

Get regular facials if possible

Keep your hands off your face

Don't:

Pick at your skin

Eat sugar

Drink sodas (regular *or* diet)

Eat fast food

Use scrubs

Use drying products

Let the phone rest on your face

Go to sleep without cleansing

Suggested Reading

Any books recommended in the chapter on sugar.

Food and Healing: How what you eat determines your health, your well-being, and the quality of your life by Annemarie Colbin (New York: Ballantine Books, 1996). I love this book. I have used it as a reference manual in my business for years. She has a wonderful cookbook I also recommend entitled *The Book of Whole Meals*.

Food & Mood: The Complete Guide to Eating Well and Feeling Your Best by Elizabeth Somer (New York: Henry Holt and Company, 1995). A good reference book chock-full of interesting information about the correlation between food and mood.

Natural Health, Natural Medicine: A Comprehensive Manual for Wellness and Self-Care by Dr. Andrew Weil (New York: Houghton Mifflin Company, 1998). I love Andrew Weil because he is an allopathic (traditional) doctor who totally recognizes the importance of the body as a whole when searching for true wellness. He has written numerous books; all of them are excellent.

6

Pregnancy & Skin Care

There are many variables that can take place with your skin during and after pregnancy. Some women don't experience any changes in their skin, while others go on a seemingly unending roller coaster ride with problem skin and breakout. There is no cure if you are one of the roller coaster riders, but there are steps you can take to help keep your skin looking its best throughout and after your pregnancy. If you're planning more than one child, once you have given birth the first time and are experienced in all the intricacies of pregnancy, your second time around will seem easier. You'll know from experience any changes occurring will usually fade away after the birth has taken place. Your body really does get back to normal—given a few inevitable transformations.

Not only can breakout be a problem while pregnant, but your skin can become photosensitive (sensitive to the sun) as well. What does this mean? The terms *chloasma, mask of pregnancy,* and *hyper-pigmentation* are all used to describe a kind of discoloration of the skin that can take place from sun exposure received while pregnant. If you are one of the unlucky women who become sensitive to the sun during this time, read further to understand the precautions you'll want to take to help keep hyperpigmentation from taking over your face.

A second concern for the new mother-to-be is the formation of stretch marks. If you are prone to this type of scarring, there is nothing short of not stretching your skin that will stop stretch marks from appearing. Whether you will get them or not is up to your genes and how much weight you gain. Although you probably can't stop them from occurring, there are treatments and creams available that can help keep your skin feeling cared for, which will be discussed later on.

A third concern for expectant mothers is having heavy, tired legs. When you are pregnant and carrying a heavier load than usual, it makes sense that your body—your legs—will feel this added weight. Incorporating stimulating treatments to invigorate tired legs can help alleviate some of the burden. These tips will be discussed later in this chapter.

All in all, the bundle of joy you are carrying around with you is the grand prize in the scheme of things. Anything your body goes through in this creative process is merely a side effect to the miracle that is taking place. But there are many things you can do in your daily routine that will have a positive effect on some of the negatives of childbearing. Let's take a look at some of these treatments.

Pregnant With Problem Skin

Hopefully you have read the previous chapter on problem skin. If not, go ahead and read through it now; then come back here for a few added tips.

The only difference between problem skin when you're expecting and when you're not is just a matter of control. When you are pregnant, your body and how it functions is essentially out of your control. I tell my clients (especially first-time pregnancies) to resign themselves to these changes. This is usually not welcome news.

Having a relaxed attitude about the changes that occur in your body—and your skin—is very important. Consider adopting The Serenity Prayer (by Reinhold Niebuhr): "God, grant me the serenity to accept the things I cannot change; courage to change the things I can; and wisdom to know the difference." When you're pregnant, serenity and wisdom will be your greatest allies. You can control your skin (raging hormones) just about as well as you can stop your belly from growing. If you realize early on that you are not in control of your body and the baby is, you will fare a whole lot better.

Case history one. A client of mine, Merry, was pregnant with her first child. Merry, then 27, had been coming to me for a little over five years. Her skin has always been clear with a few blackheads around her nose and chin along with constant slight dehydration. She has a sensitivity to sugar, but unless she has overindulged in the sweet stuff or it's "that time of the month," her skin doesn't usually breakout.

Soon after she got pregnant, her skin began to go haywire. At first she came in with mild breakout, which for her skin was unusual. As the weeks progressed, so did her breakouts until finally around the third month she basically had acne. She went from coming in for facials once a month to having one weekly. She needed all the extra help she could get.

Luckily Merry has a good head on her shoulders. She realized she couldn't really do anything about the hormones that were surging in her body. And she knew she wouldn't be able to take anything orally for the skin eruptions since she was pregnant. She decided to wait it out, hoping her skin would eventually adjust.

I had Merry on a program of constant at-home care that is the same program outlined in Chapter 5/Problem Skin. First I recommended a lot of exfoliating with a gel-type peel (gommage) to help rid the surface skin of dead cells, which could lead to more congestion. Next she used a clay mask that helped draw impurities and plugs up toward the surface and soothed her irritated skin. I also had Merry dot clay on any spots that were infected and sleep with the dots on overnight. She used a clay mask on her entire face several times per week. Exfoliating and using a clay mask were essential in keeping her skin under control—from the outside.

Geranium oil was another important addition to Merry's skin control program. It is easy to use and is essential in helping tackle problem skin. When you dot a small amount on any infected areas, the antibacterial properties in this essential oil will curb bacterial growth and help to clear the blemish without drying it out. As I've explained in the chapter on problem skin, you want to attend to the breakout with products that not only help to clear your skin, but also soothe the irritations as well. Follow the Checklist at the end of Chapter 5, but consult with your OB/GYN before using essential oils or taking any supplements listed in this book.

I am happy to say Merry's skin eventually returned to normal. It took about four months to clear up, but she no longer has any new breakout. She did have some temporary discoloration from the problem skin she experienced. Pustules and deep cysts take weeks—sometimes months—to completely clear from the skin. Even after the infection and redness is gone, the damaged tissue still has to make its way up to the surface and be sloughed off. Be patient and know that in most cases, your skin will eventually return to normal.

Case history two. Another client, Melissa, has a different kind of skin malady brought on by pregnancy. Melissa has beautiful, flawless skin. She is 38 years old, the mother of a 2-year-old son, and is 6 months pregnant. When she was pregnant with her first child, she started noticing brilliant red "dots" on her face as well as her upper chest or décolleté area. She was pretty concerned about this redness since her skin is milky white, making these dots very prominent. I assured her they were part and parcel of her pregnancy. I knew this because earlier in my career, I had gone through a total of three pregnancies with one client who developed these same red spots with every pregnancy. After each baby was born, eventually the dots disappeared.

Technically, these bright red or purplish dots are called spider angiomas, and may appear due to an excess of estrogen. They are basically dilated capillaries that look like red lines radiating from a central red dot. Once the baby is born, the hormone levels return to normal, and the dots will usually disappear on their own within three to six months.

Sure enough, about three months after Melissa gave birth to her son, the dots started to disappear. Cut to the present: pregnant again, and lo and behold, the red dots have reappeared. Now, as with so many things after the first pregnancy, Melissa has a proven history of developing these spots and the relief of knowing they do go away.

As I have said, your body is not your own during pregnancy. Things that show up in that nine-month time period many times will go away—on their own—soon after you have given birth and/ or finished breast-feeding. Remember, nothing is forever, and this includes skin irregularities developed during pregnancy. (By the way, Merry gave birth to a baby boy, Alden, and Melissa had a little girl, Kate.)

Other factors affecting your skin. When you're pregnant, your appetite is somewhat turned upside down. First you may not be able to keep food down, then you're not able to eat enough. And no doubt you will be craving many foods you don't normally eat. All of this can cause problems with your skin. This is not the time to restrict what you are eating. Do, however, try to eat a balance of healthy foods, such as the classic fruits and vegetables your body needs. Water is as important as ever along with following your doctor's prenatal vitamin regimen.

A second factor, stress, should not be overlooked as contributing to your skin problems even *after* you've given birth. Just the time factor (not having enough of it) can be a huge contributor to skin problems you may be experiencing. Trying to find anti-stress activities can help take some of the tension out of your body as well as your face.

Perhaps your grateful husband can buy you a gift certificate for a full body massage or a "day of beauty" at your favorite spa or salon. If money is an issue, go back to Chapter 2 and read the section on At-Home Facials. It talks about taking quiet time when you can, even if it's only for a few minutes. Try taking a healing bath or meditating—undisturbed—for 15 minutes.

It's really important to have time to recoup your energy. Ask your husband to take care of the baby while you draw a luxurious bubble bath, complete with candles and relaxing music. Fifteen or 30 minutes is a short amount of time for him, while for you it can make all the difference in the world. Do whatever you can to find some "me" time and recharge your batteries. Remember, anything is possible. Sometimes all you have to do is ask.

Try not to worry about the changes that may be taking place. You may not have the skin, the body, or the kind of time you had prior to your pregnancy and your child being born, but usually the body bounces back in time.

Chloasma

Chloasma is a condition also called the mask of pregnancy, hyper-pigmentation or melasma. In essence, the pigment (melanin) in your skin has gone out of control. This results in dark spots of pigmentation on the face, resembling in some cases a mask—thus the name. These are not freckles or dots, but sometimes large patches of dark brown skin commonly found on the cheeks and/or the forehead, although it is not limited to these areas.

During pregnancy or while on birth control pills ("the pill" makes your body think it's pregnant), your skin becomes photosensitive or sensitive to the sun. Photosensitivity is most common in women, especially during the childbearing years, due to fluctuating hormones. Unfortunately, if you're prone to it, the only solution for keeping chloasma away is to *stay out of the sun*. ANY amount of sun exposure will darken the pigmentation on your face. All exposure counts, and as little as a few minutes of sun can darken the spots. If you've ever experienced hyperpigmentation, you know this is true. Simple, inci-dental sun can create new spots or darken existing brown splotches on your face that may take a long time to go away. Also note that you don't have to be pregnant or on birth control pills to develop chloasma. Once you are off the pill or have given birth, you won't automatically be resistant to hyperpigmentation. You are just more *susceptible* during periods of hormonal fluctuations, but not only during these times.

Wearing sunscreen is imperative if you are experiencing any hyperpigmentation. You may want to wear sunscreen throughout your pregnancy even if you don't seem prone to pigmentation problems.

Sunscreen (discussed in detail in Chapter 10) is essential for all skins to help combat the ill effects of sun exposure. Sunscreen alone, however, will not keep hyperpigmentation away.

I tell my clients that if I had to choose between wearing sunscreen on my face without wearing a hat or wearing a hat without sunscreen, I would always—no exceptions—wear the hat without sunscreen. Why? Because it is the direct sunlight that causes damage, and in this discussion, chloasma. Although you may be wearing a sunscreen, it is only screening out or filtering the harmful UV rays. As I mention in the sun chapter later on, you want to obstruct the sun, not just filter it out. When it comes to being photosensitive, you really want to avoid direct sunlight on your face. Realistically, I would (and do) wear sunscreen *and* a hat when I'm going to be out.

Even with all the protective measures you may take, hyperpigmentation can still find a way to get to you. However, after you have given birth your hormones will usually calm down, and your skin won't be so sun sensitive. Any chloasma you may have accumulated during the pregnancy might just fade away and be gone forever. Although sometimes once you are photosensitive, you may continue to remain sensitive to the sun.

In the winter, chloasma will be less likely to develop. The sun is farther away from the earth, and the air is colder so you won't be outside as much. This doesn't mean chloasma won't announce itself, but it usually won't become as dark as in the summer time. It is in the warmer months that you really want to be careful in the sun. You will accumulate a lot more incidental sun (to and from the car, working in the garden, talking to the neighbors in the yard) without even knowing it. Any amount of exposure can darken your pigmentation; so be careful. Even if your chloasma becomes dark in the summer, it will usually fade in the winter because you'll have less outdoor activity. Just remember, chloasma won't develop or worsen unless sun exposure is involved.

Stretch Marks

I have a feeling you're hoping I'll tell you how to get rid of stretch marks or avoid them altogether. But I'm sorry to say I can't do that. Some people are predisposed genetically to the formation of stretch marks, while others may escape their plight. Like so many other things, when it comes to the body, it boils down to genetics.

Stretch marks are actually scars. As the skin of the belly is stretched during pregnancy (or weight gain in general), so too are the collagen fibers. Collagen is the supporting structure of the skin (of the dermis or inner layer). As the skin stretches to its capacity, new layers of collagen fibers are laid down to add strength to this ever-expanding tissue. This stretching action, along with the addition of new collagen, results in striae, or common stretch marks.

There are several creams on the market that claim to prevent stretch marks. They must be "miracle creams" because if you are prone to stretch marks, it will take nothing short of a miracle for your body not to produce them. Using creams and ointments on the areas that are most likely to develop stretch marks will help to keep the skin soft and supple, but it is doubtful these products will deter them from coming. If you are *not* genetically predisposed, you may not get stretch marks. It's kind of the luck of the draw, and it is predominately genetic. (What isn't?)

It's always a good idea to pay attention to areas you're concerned about. Just don't start paying a lot of money in hopes of preventing the unpreventable. But do massage your skin—all over—with creams that soothe and moisturize. Your skin will respond favorably to the care you give it. In fact, skin that is stretching tends to itch. Using moisturizers on these areas can help alleviate this side effect. Massage is an excellent way to stimulate circulation, and our skin can always use this extra boost. Maybe taking care of your expanding skin on a regular basis—before the stretch marks have begun—will actually help to minimize their appearance. It certainly can't hurt, and who knows, maybe it will really improve your chances of keeping stretch marks away.

Tired Legs

As with all maladies associated with being pregnant, nothing is going to totally eradicate them. This is also true for tired legs. But incorporating a few extra steps into your daily or weekly routine can help to relieve some of the heaviness you may be feeling.

Stimulating the circulation in your legs is the best course of treatment. A dry-brush massage (detailed in Chapter 11) is a good way to get the blood flowing through your legs. Using a body scrub in the shower is another way to invigorate your tired legs. Getting a body massage (if possible) is an excellent way to help release tension and improve blood circulation. There are massage therapists who specialize in treatments for pregnant women. Not all therapists do, but call around and see if there is someone in your area who does this kind of massage. There are even massage tables specially made for pregnant ladies. Maybe you don't want a full body massage, so just consider getting a massage on your tired legs. Or get your feet worked on. Whether you self-massage or hire someone to do the work for you, manipulating the muscles through massage is an excellent way to help relieve some of the symptoms of tired legs.

Soaking in Epsom salts can temporarily lessen the tired feeling in your legs, but consult with your doctor to be sure you can add products to your bathwater. Although extremely hot baths and whirlpools are not recommended (you can sweat to regulate your body temperature, but the baby can't), relaxing in a warm tub of water with soothing salts or essences can help improve the circulation in your legs and bring you relief.

There are products on the market made specifically to help tired, heavy legs. They may contain essential oils and/or other ingredients to help stimulate and improve circulation. You may want to try some of these and see if they make a difference.

Finally, sometimes just elevating your legs can help with some of the discomfort. It can help to get the blood away from your feet where it tends to pool. Taking the load off your tired, swollen legs can go a long way in helping them feel better. It's a simple remedy, but it can really bring relief.

Out Of Time

When you have an infant to take care of, you're lucky if you can brush your teeth. Forget about your skin! I hear this complaint over and over from new mothers. It seems there just isn't any time to take care of yourself, your skin included. So adopting a new attitude is probably in order. This attitude is similar to the Zen imagery of being a rock in the stream. You can fight against the water coming down around you, or you can just sit in the stream and enjoy the shower you are experiencing. "Go with the flow" is a more concise way of putting it.

The first few months after the birth of your child, you probably won't have time to do much. If you can brush your teeth, however, you can cleanse your face. When going to brush, take a few extra *seconds* and grab your cleanser. Put it on your face, brush your teeth, rinse the cleanser off, and you're practically done. After rinsing the cleanser off and drying your face, spray your face with toner. (If you followed my suggestion in Chapter 1, you already have your toner in a spray bottle.) The only thing left is moisturizer. A few more seconds will get it on your face, and you have accomplished the impossible: you have completed your Basic 1-2-3 program in record time! It literally only takes a few extra seconds to wash, spray toner, and apply some cream to your face. Without this twice-a-day care, your skin may be headed for trouble. It will take you two minutes, *tops*, to do The Basics, morning and night.

I never expect new moms to do their weekly exfoliating and masking. I just assume this is "mission impossible." But in case you are one of the lucky ones with a few extra minutes once or twice a week, read over Chapter 2. These two steps (exfoliating and using a clay mask) will help you maintain healthy, clean skin. If you cannot see your way clear to taking this extra time, keep it in mind in case you do have more time later on. The most important steps for your skin are The Basics 1-2-3. The Extras are just that, and at this point do what you can, when you can, and don't worry about the rest. You've got a lot of other things to attend to—namely your new bundle of joy.

Getting a facial every month or every 6-8 weeks would be an enormous gift. In the capable hands of a professional, you can help to undo weeks of neglect that have built up in your skin. By no means are facials going to miraculously reverse problems that may have occurred, but they can further the health of your skin tremendously. Plus for that hour in the treatment room, you can get away completely and luxuriate without worrying about the baby crying or the telephone ringing.

The bottom line, don't stress yourself out about not being able to take great care of your skin. After your baby gets into a rhythm, so will your life (sort of), and you will probably find more chunks of time to accomplish tasks for yourself. Enjoy your new baby, and do what you can for yourself. Breathe, relax when you can, and know that you have created a living miracle. I suppose the next miracle is to find time for the miracle worker—you!

7

Men & Skin *I have written this especially for men.*

There really is very little difference between treating male skin and treating female skin. I approach each person as a unique individual—male, female, black, white, young, or old. Everyone has several combinations of characteristics that make up his or her skin. There are, of course, certain qualities to men's skin that make it distinct. Dare I say, when it comes to skin care, the main difference between men and women is apathy. You—generally—don't pay much attention to your skin. I don't think this is because you don't care. It's often a matter of exposure (or lack of). Classically you are not exposed to proper skin care techniques (and products) the way women are throughout their lives. That is changing, and consequently I see many more men taking good care of their skin.

Your skin care program is basically the same as for women: The Basics 1-2-3 (Chapter 1) morning and night as well as The Extras (Chapter 2) at least once a week. If you have problems with breakout, read through Chapter 5/Problem Skin.

Your skin is usually thick; thick skin tends to be oily. You have high amounts of androgens, including testosterone (a male hormone linked to sebaceous activity), so your skin will usually be oilier than a woman's. You typically experience problems with your skin at the onset of puberty, when your body is going through tremendous hormonal surges. Along with blemishes, you may experience irritations due to your newly sprouting facial hair.

Also many young men are active in sports at this time. Sweating during these activities can bring its own set of problems—namely irritation on the surface of the skin. Couple this irritation with chin straps or other gear that may interfere with sweating, and you have a recipe for trouble.

After puberty, you generally don't have too many problems with your skin. As apposed to women, who have monthly hormone fluctuations throughout their lives, many of you have smooth sailing after the teen years. This, however, is not always the case.

Do you have problems with your skin? If so, you might have a **hormone imbalance** that can cause mild to severe breakouts. **Folliculitis** (discussed later) and basic irritation with shaving can plague you throughout your life too. **Diet** also plays a key role in the health of your skin. An overall **lack of proper care** can cause problems as well. If neglected, your skin will reflect it.

One common problem you may experience is **extreme dryness** (which is really dehydration) that comes from a lack of moisture in the skin as well as a thick dead skin buildup. Exfoliating and moisturizing can help lessen this type of red, flaky skin. However, dry skin may actually be eczema, a dermatitis showing up as red, scaly skin that usually itches. In this case, skin care products will not be of much help, and you'll want to seek out a dermatologist's care.

Sun damage is another skin problem I see frequently in my male clients. Because you're not as conscious about taking care of your skin as women are, you tend to skip sunscreen and sun protection in general. This can lead to sunburn as well as general dryness (dehydration) from overexposure. Whenever sun exposure is involved, there is always the possibility of cancerous growths down the road. As with all skin, female *and* male, sun protection is a must. See Chapter 12 (The Forgotten Places) for special consideration of those areas that get a lot of sun, as well as Chapter 10, which discusses the sun in detail.

A common condition for men is **ingrown hairs**, otherwise known as pseudofolliculitis barbae. This is where your hair decides to navigate back down into the skin instead of coming out onto the surface. Because these hairs are coarse, they can wreak havoc on the tissue below. They usually cause red, irritated bumps that resemble blemishes; but they are actually small irritations caused by the ingrown hairs. Once this sensitive tissue meets with a razor, small red bumps (razor bumps) follow. Although ingrown hairs cause inflammation and irritation, there is usually not a bacterial infection present as with true folliculitis.

Pseudofolliculitis tends to happen more with curly-haired men, especially African-Americans. The first course of treatment for ingrown hairs is exfoliation. By exfoliating the outer, dead skin layer, often the hair finds an easier path to the outside. When exfoliating, a gel-type, nonabrasive peel would be preferable to using a scrub. (See Chapter 2/Exfoliation: What to use.) If a scrub is all you have at the moment, don't get too aggressive with it or you can cause more irritation, but be on the lookout for a gentler, gel-type product. Give exfoliation a try and see if it solves your ingrown hair problems. If you can, try not shaving so closely with your razor. This can help to alleviate some of the irritation. If nothing seems to work, another option—although maybe not for everyone—is to let your beard grow out.

If you're having problems with skin irritations around your beard area that won't go away, it could be true folliculitis. This is a bacterial infection (staphylococcus) in your hair follicles caused by any number of things, even contaminated washcloths. If you think you have folliculitis, you may want to consult your dermatologist, who can prescribe topical or oral antibiotics to get rid of the bacteria present in your skin.

The following is *one* profile of how some of you take care of your skin. I know this is a generalization, but it is based on seeing male clients over the years, listening to stories about my female clients' husbands, and asking men wherever I go how they take care of their skin. I know there are those of you (more and more) who are conscientious about your skin and who really do have good skin care habits. The following is not a profile of *you*, but of "the others."

You almost always use soap. And you use the same soap on your face as you do on your body—whatever is within reach in the shower. This can include deodorant soaps, which by the way, are working to inhibit the sweat glands from producing. How can this be good for your face? After washing with soap in the shower, you usually shave. Next you use aftershave. Many times these products contain alcohol. Sometimes you slap on a moisturizer (any one will do), and you're off. That's it—simple, easy, done. You may only use soap in the shower and never mess with moisturizer or even an aftershave. Your reasoning is, "What for?" You aren't having any problems with your skin, so why bother with products? At night, sometimes you just splash your face with water.

Believe me, I'm not advocating men following a complicated skin care routine (women either) when the less-is-more approach seems to be working just fine. I am, however, suggesting incorporating a few minor changes that would be beneficial. The following is a condensed version of the skin care program introduced in Chapters 1 and 2.

Don't use deodorant soaps. They inhibit the natural eliminating process (sweating) and can cause serious irritation, not to mention the drying effect soap can have on your skin. All soaps, deodorant or not, are generally alkaline, and you want to use products that are acidic or at least non-alkaline. A foaming gel or milky, non-alkaline cleanser is your best bet. (See Chapter 1/Cleansing: What to use.)

Use toner/aftershave *without alcohol*. Products with alcohol will just dry out the surface of your skin and may cause burning or irritation if applied after shaving. Using an appropriate toner can actually soothe the skin after you shave, which is what your skin needs. I recommend putting your toner in a spray bottle (see Chapter 1/Toning: How to use toner), which makes it easy to spray on as an aftershave. Be sure to include your whole face and neck when spraying. Toner is a quick and easy way to help calm, soothe, and reacidify your skin.

Use moisturizer made for the face. Keeping the skin well hydrated helps keep your outer, dead skin soft, which might also help keep you from getting ingrown hairs. Moisturizers protect your skin from the environment and keep you from feeling dry. Many of you don't think you need a moisturizer. Perhaps this is because you are so used to the way your skin feels without one. If you're not currently using a moisturizer, try one and see how it feels. Use a cream formulated for the face instead of a body lotion. Make sure to find products that are made for your particular skin type as well (see Chapter 4). Even if you have problems with oil, find a light-textured cream or gel moisturizer formulated for oily skin. Gels will feel as though you don't have anything on while moisturizing your skin.

Exfoliate. Every time you shave you are, in essence, exfoliating the skin where your beard grows. It is important, however, to exfoliate your whole face to keep the dead skin buildup to a minimum. This will not only keep your skin feeling smooth, it will help to keep breakouts and ingrown hairs to a minimum. Whether you have problem skin or not, exfoliation is an important step for overall skin care maintenance.

Sunscreen is a must. Most of you tend to skip this very important step. I can't stress enough the importance of avoiding sun damage; therefore, wearing sunscreen is essential. Wear it whenever you're going to be outside. Don't forget the tops of your ears. This is where I see a lot of sun damage on men. Even if you wear a baseball cap when running, golfing, sailing, or whatever outside activity you're engaged in, your ears are still constantly exposed to the sun. So don't forget to put some sunscreen there.

The same need for sun protection applies to balding heads. Many times I have seen a follicularly challenged man driving around, no hat, with the top down on his convertible. This can prove to be disastrous given time. Remember, sun exposure is sun exposure whether you're at the beach or sitting in your convertible. The sun will damage whoever is bold enough to go outside unprotected. (See Chapter 12/Balding heads.)

Professional care. More and more of you are getting facials. The stigma against skin care for men is finally abating. Why is a man getting a facial any different than a woman getting one? You get haircuts and massages just like women do. Why not facials?

Maybe you associate facials with makeup and cosmetics. Perhaps you picture Dorothy (from the *Wizard of Oz*) being worked over from head to toe, having her hair and nails done while someone else is applying makeup. I assure you, this is not what facials are all about. As described in Chapter 3, facials are professional treatments meant to help the skin on many different levels. Anyone who has skin can benefit from having a facial.

There are some skin care salons that cater to a female clientele. And I can understand why you might feel a bit uncomfortable and out of place in one of those facilities. But just like gyms that are unisex, there are facial salons (most, actually) that welcome men too.

Most of the men I've given facials to have really enjoyed them— sometimes much to their own surprise. They all comment on how relaxing a facial is. I'm not sure what they were expecting, but they all leave with a different, more accepting outlook on having skin care treatments.

I encourage you to give facials a try. They can go a long way in easing the tension out of your face, keeping your skin clean, smooth, and free from problems as well as helping you relax, which is always welcome.

Quick Tips

- Almost without exception, the men I have given facials to fall into a deep sleep during the course of an hour-long treatment. Why not get a facial during lunch time? You can catch a good, long nap and come out with better skin in the process.
- Usually men are turned off to skin care products because of their fragrances. But there are products on the market that are made specifically for men and therefore don't smell too perfumed.

8

Determining Products

Listening to my clients over the years, there seems to be a pattern a lot of people follow: you try a product line, having been seduced by the claim of perfect skin or anti-aging abilities; you invest a lot of money in these miracles in a jar; and you wait for the miraculous results that never come. Initially, you see an improvement in your skin. It glows or clears up temporarily, and you think you've found the answer to your skin care woes. After a few months, the results start fading away, and you're faced with the same skin you had before you started this miracle regimen. So you go back to the land of products, usually the department store, and search once again for another product line that claims to produce amazing results. And the cycle continues.

The truth is, it's hard to find products that work. Considering the number of skin care lines available, you would think a large percentage of them would be effective. Unfortunately for the unknowing consumer, there are many products that are fairly ineffective. The advertisements might have you believing otherwise, but the sad truth is there is a lot of mediocrity in skin care. You will have to go through a trial and error period with different product lines before you find one that works for you. One product line may work well with your skin, and another may not. This depends on the current condition of your skin, the climate where you live, what your diet consists of, and your skin type. Because of all these factors, I did not include specific product recommendations in this book. However, I would be more than happy to discuss your skin care needs with you. Information on contacting me can be found at the back of the book.

Whenever possible, I go to the department store and "cruise" the beauty section. As I approach the counter, I am greeted immediately by various salespeople eager to show me the latest miracle in their skin care line—sometimes donning white lab coats, usually wearing inch-thick makeup (covering their skin). I feel as though I have been descended upon by sales-hungry piranha. I start by asking basic questions about ingredients and how the products work. It is at this point their special sales techniques kick in, but they usually can't come up with reasonable answers to my basic questions. What I tend to hear is a bunch of sales and skin care mumbo-jumbo. As I probe deeper and ask more complex questions, it is clear these sales people truly *are* experts in their field—which is sales. If the answer isn't in their "script," they are caught off guard, referring back to their selling points. Once in a while I will be surprised by some intelligent (and accurate) answers, but more often than not, the department store's cosmetic salesperson fails miserably to make any real sense.

I believe the reason for their inability to answer my questions is twofold. As I've already said, their knowledge of the skin is limited to what they have learned from the product line they work for. But more importantly when caring for the skin, there are no miracles. Many products make outrageous claims, and the truth is these claims usually don't hold up. Most products simply cannot produce the results their ads want you to believe. Trying to sell a miracle in a jar where miracles don't exist is a tough job for anyone—expert or not.

So keep in mind there are no miracles that can dramatically change your skin overnight. Proper and consistent care is the key to healthy skin. Generally, even products with well-worded ad campaigns cannot instantly change your skin's condition. Nor can they erase a lifetime of neglect or problem skin. It's a harsh reality perhaps, but going into the department store or anywhere products are sold with this knowledge will save you a lot of money and disappointment.

You may not be aware that there are two different classifications for products in the skin care industry: retail and professional. Read further to get familiar with all of your options so you can be a smart shopper when it comes time to buy skin care products.

Retail Products

Retail products are sold in a retail environment, like a department or grocery store. These products are sold to the mass market. Manufacturers annually spend millions of dollars for ad campaigns on TV and in magazines, enticing you to buy their products. A retail environment is usually where the average consumer looks to purchase skin care products.

Most people look to the department store not only to purchase skin care products, but to get their skin care advice as well. Many consumers just don't know where else to turn. Retail, department store products are sold by counter salespeople who generally have no hands-on experience with skin. They go through product training pertaining to the line they are selling, but usually lack any practical experience in treating skin. If you have no-problem skin, you will probably fare reasonably well in the department store because not a lot will be required from either the products or the sales staff. But if you have problems with your skin (or just want professional skin care advice), I recommend talking to a licensed aesthetician. Not all professionals excel at their craft, but at least they have training and a license to back up what they are saying.

Other retail products are sold in drug or grocery stores. In this case, you are on your own. There is no salesperson to help (or pressure) you. At the grocery store you can take your time, read labels at your leisure, and really study the products before you buy. Many times you will pay premium prices at the department store for comparable products found at the local grocery, paying for name brands in fancy bottles and their ads with beautiful models. Products at the drug or grocery store may not have great packaging and are not marketed as aggressively, but their prices reflect this.

Finally, there are the multilevel, marketing-type products, again sold by salespeople, not skin care professionals. They are trained on the product, not specifically on skin. I'm not saying that everyone who isn't a professional aesthetician is unqualified to help you with your skin, I only recommend you look closely at the people who are giving you advice. What does *their* skin look like? And most importantly, are they making sense—or just a sale?

In general, retail products tend to be fairly inactive, rendering them less effective in their ability to tackle specific skin problems. This is the dilemma with retail products. They can't really afford to be very potent or the products would no doubt be returned en masse. Even a great product can cause problems if the skin is misdiagnosed and an inappropriate product is recommended and used. What you may find with retail products is skin care advice from a salesperson plus products that do very little for your skin.

Professional Products

Professional products are sold exclusively in a salon or spa by a licensed aesthetician. The idea being that a professional can correctly diagnose your skin and recommend appropriate products. In this professional setting, the aesthetician can take care of your skin on an ongoing basis, both through facial treatments as well as with products.

In the professional realm, there is a great separation between retail and professional products. For instance, I would never consider using or selling a retail product (something you could find at any department store for example) in my office. Why? Quite simply, quality. Professional products are invariably superior in quality to their retail counterparts—not always, but usually. Professional products can address specific needs, whereas retail products are more general or generic.

Couperose skin (see Chapter 4 for a detailed description) is one of the best examples of this. I would be hard-pressed to find a retail product specifically made to address this common skin care problem, whereas many professional lines do. In fact, I'm sure I would have a difficult time finding a retail salesperson who could explain what couperose is, let alone have a product to recommend. The quality of the product as well as its ability to address specific skin care needs are two areas that separate professional from retail.

In almost every professional line there are specialized products that are produced exclusively for use in a facial by a professional. These products are generally not available for the consumer to purchase. Retail products are ordinarily made solely for at-home use. Occasionally you will find retail products being used in a professional environment, usually at department store day spas or salons. Using a retail product in a professional environment (in facial treatments) would be extremely limiting. Again, there wouldn't be the class of products required to address a client with special needs.

Unfortunately, not all professional products are going to give you great results. With the myriad of products available to you (retail *and* professional), very few will truly meet your needs. Many clients come to me discouraged, having jumped from one product to another, never finding anything that truly works for them. But take heart, exceptional products do exist. It may just take time to find them.

Determining A Good Product

There is no magical way to know if a particular product or product line is good. The determining factor will always be: how does it make your skin look and feel? I used to say ingredients were everything. Now I look at the product's effectiveness as a whole as well as what it's made of. But the ingredient list is always the first thing I look at when analyzing a product. You want an ingredient list you can read and comprehend. Is it all synthetic—using long, chemical names? Or are the ingredients identifiable? An ingredient list should have some recognizable, everyday words like *sunflower seed oil* or *chamomile extract*, etc. Not all complex words mean an ingredient is synthetic (for instance, vitamin E may be listed as *tocopheryl acetate*), but if the entire list is unrecognizable, it's probably a synthetic product.

What's wrong with synthetic? When you get right down to it, everything on earth consists of chemicals. Synthetics are made up of molecules of chemicals, just like organic or natural substances. But synthetic products are usually inert, meaning they are not active. Synthetic products are basically composed of inorganic, laboratory-made ingredients, which are synthetic—fake. Organic, natural, or active products are made from natural sources like plants, fruits, and vegetal oils. The difference between synthetic and organic is best depicted by using essential oils. I discuss these natural essences in detail later in this chapter, but for now I will use them to illustrate my point.

Pure essential oils are very powerful. These essences contain many chemical constituents that render them active even after they are extracted from their plant sources. Natural essential oils are acidic on the pH scale and have an inherent medicinal benefit on the skin's surface. Inorganic or synthetic essential oils are made in a chemist's lab of similar molecules. Their chemical makeup may be alike, but chemists cannot put the "life force" into their laboratory creations. It is this life force that will constitute the effectiveness of the product. These synthetic copies may smell reminiscent of their organic siblings, but they are not exact. Synthetics can only mimic the real thing. And when it comes to ingredients used on the skin, I recommend the real thing. Your skin is a living entity, and I believe it will respond to real, organic products over synthetics.

When looking for products, I recommend looking for ingredients that connote real substances with organic matter employed. Although synthetic ingredients aren't necessarily *bad* for your skin (they usually won't cause flare-ups or irritations), they can't help to soothe or otherwise stimulate the skin. Organic ingredients, on the other hand, can be both soothing and stimulating. One last point—synthetic products tend to be void of smell. Natural or organic products usually have wonderful aromatics based on the botanical ingredients used.

I look for organic ingredients, or at least *predominantly* organic, in the professional products I use. Absolutely pure products are hard to find, but I have come across a few all-natural, professional products over the years. Although the ingredient list is impressive, the products may have some built-in problems. If they are entirely organic, common chemical preservatives (like methylparaben and propylparaben) are not used, and the products can become unstable. They will have a much shorter shelf life, and bacteria from the air will affect and many times contaminate them. There may be a problem with consistency as well. The organic matter will change with different weather conditions and crop harvests, and therefore, so will the manufactured product. It's hard to continually crank out an all-natural product consistent with the former batch. All-natural products tend to be quite expensive as well. Finding a product that is *predominately* natural is a good idea, but if completely natural is what you prefer, you may run into some of the problems mentioned above.

Quick Tips

- Beware of a product that is a moisturizer *and* a sunscreen *and* foundation, or any other combination of actions. The more feats a product claims to carry out, the more ingredients it will require, and it will be more likely to cause sensitivities.
- Burning and/or itching is always a cause for concern. Products that are right for your skin will feel good and not cause irritations.
- Department store products require a lot of money for advertising and marketing. Many times what you end up with is expensive, grocery store-quality products with pretty packaging and famous models as spokespeople.

Essential Oils

I want to discuss essential oils as ingredients since they have so many beneficial actions on the skin. I have been using products with these natural essences in them for over a dozen years. Their effectiveness is powerful, and I have many clients who have turned their skin around through the use of essential oils.

What are essential oils? They are aromatic liquids that are found in certain plants and flowers. Essential oils are fragrant essences that are produced in specialized glands within the plant as part of the process of photosynthesis. Essential oils are volatile, like gases, and have a very thin viscosity—similar to water. (Actually, essential oils, by definition, are volatile. Fatty oils are termed *fixed*.) If you put a drop of pure essential oil on your skin, it will evaporate almost immediately, whereas any fatty oil (like avocado, wheat germ, or mineral oil) will remain on the surface with little penetration.

Essential oils are lighter than water, so they float on the surface and therefore were thought of as oils as far back as Cleopatra's time. They are not, however, fatty oils. When I talk about essential oils, people with oily skin start getting nervous. They fear their skin will break out once they use products with so many "oils" in them. I understand the word *oil* to a person with oily skin has a negative connotation, but essential oils aren't like regular oils. In many cases essential oils can help *reduce* the amount of oil produced by the sebaceous glands.

Essential oils are antiseptic and antibacterial. They are perfect for problem skin, adding antibacterial properties to products without adding extra oils. Essential oils are stimulating to the circulation. Since your skin cells are nourished by the oxygen and nutrients carried in the blood, any circulatory benefits are always welcomed. These aromatic essences are oxygenating and detoxifying and have a positive effect on the capillaries. Essential oils are also acidic, thus complementing the acidic nature of the skin.

Just because a product says it contains essential oils doesn't mean it is a good product. It will depend on the percentage of aromatic essences, the grade or quality of the oils, and the ingredients the essential oils are surrounded by. Even though a product claims to contain essential oils, don't stop investigating.

One surefire way to know if the products you're using contain pure essential oils is to look at the packaging. Pure oils cannot be housed in plastic; they have to be in either glass or metal containers. If a product claiming to contain essential oils comes in a plastic jar or tube, most likely it does not contain pure oils or it has a low percentage of oils. There are hybrid plastics in use by some companies that are said to be sound for housing essential oils. But as a general rule, if you see products in plastic, they don't contain pure essential oils.

Another telltale sign of the purity of essential oils is price. The average consumer isn't going to be up on the prices for different oils, but here are a few examples. Each individual plant source has its own particular way in which the essential oil is extracted. Usually the choices are steam distillation, maceration, dissolving (using a volatile solvent), and pressing. Essential oil of rose is one of the most expensive essential oils on the market. Why? Rose oil is commonly obtained through steam distillation of the petals and sometimes the stamens as well. It takes five *tons* of rose petals to extract 2 1/4 *pounds* of essential oil! Now you can see why rose oil is so expensive. If you purchase a product that says it contains rose oil, it will have to be expensive, or it is using adulterated or synthetic oil. Lavender oil, in comparison to rose oil, is relatively inexpensive to manufacture. It is also acquired through steam distillation. It takes approximately 220 pounds of lavender flowers to procure two pounds of essential oil.

Unless you know the ins and outs of essential oils and how they are individually priced, you won't necessarily be able to tell if you're buying adulterated oils or not. My point in telling you about the prices is to simply alert you to the fact that pure essential oils aren't cheap. If a product (especially a retail, mass marketed product) says it contains large quantities of many essential oils, you may not be getting the real thing. It's a complex subject, and there are many wonderful books written about aromatherapy (the science of essential oils) and essential oils themselves. If you're really curious, you may be interested in reading further on this topic. (See Suggested Reading.)

One of the side benefits of using essential oils is their wonderful aromatics. It's not really a side benefit because how things smell will affect you on many levels. Because of the intense aromatic qualities of essential oils, using products that contain them can be an olfactory pleasure all day long.

I don't recommend that you play around with essential oils. Nor do I suggest you mix them into your face products. They are very potent substances and can cause serious irritations and/or injury to the skin if not used properly. Find a product line that employs essential oils and rely on the manufacturer's expertise to create a beneficial aromatherapy product.

Aromatherapy is very big today, so it's not hard to find products that contain essential oils. You still want to ask a lot of questions and try the product out before you buy if possible. An ingredient list that has essential oils in it doesn't necessarily reflect the effectiveness of the actual product. Experiment and give products with essential oils a try. I think you will find they are truly, unforgettably wonderful.

Suggested Reading

Aromatherapy: A Holistic Guide by Ann Berwick (St. Paul, Minnesota: Llewellyn Publications, 1997) is a well-rounded book all about the art, science, and application of essential oils. It makes for a very good read.

Aromatherapy, An A—Z by Patricia Davis (Essex, England: The C.W. Daniel Company Limited, 1995) is a great reference guide in dictionary form for aromatherapy, individual essential oils, and conditions helped through the use of essential oils.

Aromatherapy: The Complete Guide to Plant & Flower Essences for Health & Beauty by Daniele Ryman (New York: Bantam Books, 1993). This is another excellent book by one of the most respected authorities on aromatherapy.

The Complete Book of Essential Oils & Aromatherapy by Valerie Ann Worwood (San Rafael, California: New World Library, 1991) is a classic encyclopedic book with every conceivable use for essential oils and aromatherapy in daily life. It contains numerous recipes for using these medicinal, botanical extracts.

Trends & Fads

The following products and procedures are some of the many ways available for fighting the aging process. Some of them may indeed bring you the desired results, while others may give you a negligible payoff and possibly put a large dent in your pocketbook. As you will read in Chapter 17, I am not a proponent of dramatically changing the appearance you were blessed with. However, there are many ways that you can do this if you are so inclined. I recommend reading as much as you can about any new miracle treatment before you decide to indulge in it. Since there are new products and procedures coming out almost daily, I have tried to include those that are the most popular today.

Alpha Hydroxy Acids (AHAs)

What are AHAs? Exfoliating is the most important thing you can do for your skin. Getting rid of the mounting dead cell layers will go a long way to restoring and maintaining healthy skin. Exfoliation gives your skin more clarity, cleaner pores, and a much smoother texture. Alpha hydroxy acids are one way to achieve this well-exfoliated surface.

Alpha hydroxy acids, or AHAs, dissolve the intercellular cement that binds your skin cells together. These acids essentially loosen the glue between the cells, allowing them to slough off more readily. This creates smoother skin, steps up circulation, and can lessen the lines caused from dehydration. I'm referring to superficial lines—not deep wrinkles. The results vary, but in general you should experience an improvement in the texture of your skin with the use of AHAs. They really can make the surface of your skin incredibly smooth, which helps with the dehydrated (dry) feeling that is so common. You may also experience less debris clogging your pores after using AHA products. I have seen this type of improvement in some of my clients with chronic congestion problems.

Alpha hydroxy acids are sometimes termed *fruit acids* since several of the acids come from fruit sources. There are many different kinds of AHAs available for use in skin care products. Some of these acids are glycolic, derived from sugarcane; lactic, from sour milk and other sources such as bilberry or passion fruit; tartaric, from grapes and aged wine; and citric, from citrus fruits such as lemon and orange.

AHAs are what I term *passive exfoliators*. Just by the mere fact that they are sitting on your skin, they are helping to decompose cells, leading to a smoother texture. But it is my belief you still need to *actively* exfoliate (with a gommage or scrub) on a regular basis to get the optimum effects from passive exfoliation. In doing so, you help to eliminate much more of the buildup that the AHAs have broken down. For example, let's say you pour paint thinner (AHAs) on a sidewalk (your skin) covered with paint (dead skin cells). The paint thinner dissolves and breaks up a lot of the paint, but until you get a hose and really blast the sidewalk with a powerful stream of water (an active exfoliator), the decomposed paint just sits there. Putting AHAs on your skin helps to decompose skin cells, but until you actively exfoliate, you are only doing half the job—and only receiving half the results.

If you are prone to couperose (capillary damage) or if you have sensitive skin, be careful with AHAs. Their acidic nature makes them an irritant, which can cause a mild to strong burning sensation on skin that is sensitive. I have found AHAs also heighten redness in my clients with couperose. In some cases where the AHAs are really helping to unclog pores, the payoff is greater than the slight redness it may be causing. Just be aware AHAs can cause further damage to the fragile capillaries. If you continue to feel a stinging or burning sensation when using AHAs, I'd take the hint and stop using them. As prevalent as alpha hydroxy acids are, they are not for everyone. Listen to the clues your skin is giving you.

Something else that is a point of concern is the use of "mono acids" (meaning one). Glycolic is probably the most commonly used mono alpha hydroxy acid. When you continue to use an acidic compound over a long period of time (especially in high strengths) thinking that if a little is good then more is even better, it can be too severe for your skin to tolerate. Your skin can become irritated, which in turn can cause edema (water retention or puffiness). This reaction can cause a negative breakdown of healthy tissue, not just the decomposing of surface dead cells. There are companies who recognize this dilemma and are putting out multiacid AHA products. Using multiple acid formulas is preferable to mono acid products because you are utilizing acid compounds from several sources instead of just one. In the long run, the skin will react better to this variety.

How strong is too strong? Lower-strength (3% or less) AHA compounds do not present a threat to the health of your skin and can be used daily without concern. When using high-strength AHAs (10% or more), it is much better to use them on a semiregular basis rather than using them every day. Again, high-strength products can become too much of a good thing.

Many AHAs on the market—especially glycolics—are synthetic. One of the large chemical companies here in the U.S. produces most commercial-grade glycolic. The technology was first developed for glycolic acid to be produced from sugarcane, its organic source. Then synthetics were substituted. My personal preference is organic over synthetic. You get the whole synergistic effect of the natural extract instead of an imitation. If the AHAs in a product come from organic sources, most likely they will state that on the ingredient list.

Another thing you may have heard about is BHAs, or beta hydroxy acids. The basic difference between AHAs and BHAs is this: AHAs dissolve intercellular cement—the gluelike substance that binds cells together. BHAs break down the cells themselves. Betas dissolve dead tissue with a protein-dissolving action similar to enzymes, like papaya and bromaline (from pineapple). Salicylic acid, for instance, is a beta hydroxy acid derived from willow bark.

Compared to many of the trends and fads on the market today that are of no benefit, I think AHAs and BHAs are actually beneficial. They're not for everybody, but they can give you good results without incurring too much, if any, damage. The premise behind many of the products and procedures in skin care is to exfoliate the skin, and alpha hydroxy acids deliver. They aren't the be-all and end-all, and they certainly don't take the place of actively exfoliating and deep cleansing your skin as recommended in Chapter 2, but AHAs can smooth your complexion and help keep your pores from clogging as well as providing your skin with a healthy, radiant appearance.

Bo-Tox®

What is Bo-Tox? I call this "Magic Poison." And essentially, that is exactly what Bo-Tox is. It is actually the botulism bacterium (botulism toxin) that is injected into specific areas of the face, usually the forehead and between the eyebrows. The poison renders the surrounding muscles paralyzed. Once the site is injected and the muscles are paralyzed, you are unable to express or move that area of your face. Without daily and constant expressing, lines do not furrow into the skin. So Bo-Tox, by paralyzing the muscles, indirectly helps to reduce the deepening of wrinkles. It lasts four to six months and has to be reinjected to continue the benefits.

Bo-Tox has been used for years to help stop eye tics and other medical maladies. It has just recently been "discovered" for its anti-aging, cosmetic benefits. It still has not been approved by the FDA for cosmetic use. It is only administered by a licensed doctor, either a dermatologist or a plastic surgeon.

One client's story. Recently I had sent my client Barbara to see her dermatologist about a mole I was concerned about. She is 47 years old and has beautiful skin that has very few lines. Barbara truly has the skin of a woman in her mid-30s. During her last facial, she told me about her trip to the dermatologist. Luckily the mole wasn't anything to worry about, but I found what happened later on somewhat disturbing.

The dermatologist asked Barbara to frown in order to furrow her brow, and she gladly obliged. He proceeded to tell her he could inject her "worry lines" (lines that form between the eyebrows) with Bo-Tox. Ask anyone to form a line of expression, and guess what you'll get? A line of expression—a wrinkle. So there she was, feeling like something was wrong with her face, and the solution was being conveniently presented to her in the form of a quick-fix injection.

It was such a blatant, bold-faced way to make her feel ill at ease and to endorse the sale of his services. Plus his comments were unsolicited. She was going in to get a mole checked, not to inquire about anti-aging procedures. Even if Barbara had deep worry lines, I still wouldn't defend this ploy by her dermatologist.

My point in retelling this story is to instill an air of caution in you if and when you find yourself in a similar circumstance. Don't fall prey to someone else's opinion of how you should look, especially when the opinion-giver stands to gain $300-$500 for one injection of Bo-Tox (or any other corrective procedure). Remember the saying "Let the buyer beware!"

Collagen Injections

What are collagen injections? This is a procedure where bovine collagen, taken from cowhide, is injected into the furrows of deep lines and wrinkles of the face. The most commonly injected areas are the nasolabial lines (laugh lines), fine lines around the lips and corners of the mouth, and the vertical lines between the eyebrows (worry lines).

The collagen acts like a filler to plump up the depression caused by a wrinkle, making the line (wrinkle) temporarily disappear. The actual procedure will cause redness in the injected area along with temporary bruising and a bit of swelling. These minor reactions will usually go away within the first 24 hours.

In all of the literature written about collagen injections, two main points are repeated. First, collagen injections are a quick and easy "fix." This procedure will give you the fastest results with a minimum of complications. However, it also is a very short-lived fix, and you have to be reinjected frequently to continue the results.

The price of collagen varies from doctor to doctor, but one syringeful costs from $300-$500. Since you have to constantly repeat this procedure to maintain the benefits, collagen treatments can get quite costly. Three to nine months is the life span of collagen injected into the skin. It is reabsorbed at varying speeds, but as much as 30% is reabsorbed within the first three months after the injection.

In addition to the high cost, there is another problem—the potential for allergic reactions. Around 3% of the general public is allergic to bovine collagen. I've read that if you have an intolerance to beef and other bovine products, you will most likely have a reaction to cow collagen. Therefore, before having collagen injected for cosmetic purposes, you will always be tested for allergic reactions. Usually the collagen test is in the forearm, and sometimes it's behind the hairline, on the scalp. A second, follow-up test is standard practice with many doctors—just in case you have a delayed reaction to the first test. This precaution is taken because experiencing an allergic reaction to collagen would be disastrous!

If you are allergic to cowhide collagen or you just don't want the bovine experience, you can use your body's own collagen, which is called autologous collagen. Surgery is required to obtain this type of collagen, usually from the upper thighs or buttocks. The potential problem is that if you continue to get regular treatments with autologous collagen, more of your collagen will need to be donated. This requires more surgery to transplant, then more injections into your wrinkles. In the long run, is it worth all the trouble?

Collagen injections should only be administered by a licensed doctor, usually a dermatologist or plastic surgeon. You want to make sure to find a doctor who does a lot of these injections. Accuracy is imperative for proper results.

Glycolic Peels

What are glycolic peels? I am not a proponent of glycolic peels. I realize they are popular, but once again I find myself going against the grain. Glycolic peels usually come in a series of six treatments. What is magical about six? My guess would be money and not so much a technical result. Many times the series is given in one-week increments. My belief is that if you had a good facial once a week for six weeks, your skin would look just as fabulous without using harsh acid peels.

Strong peels, using glycolic or other alpha hydroxy acids, will decompose surface cells. Glycolic acid also causes the capillaries to dilate, which brings more blood to the area. Blood carries oxygen and other nutrients to feed and nourish the skin cells. So far, so good. But glycolic acid can also weaken the capillaries. The hot sensation you feel with the application of a strong glycolic peel is the intense dilation of your capillaries coupled with the acid that is decomposing dead cells. It is this excessive dilating that creates a consequence that far outweighs any oxygenating and exfoliating benefits you may receive. Because capillaries are naturally weak, strong dilating can cause capillary damage or couperose. Couperose, as discussed in Chapter 4, is a condition that rarely improves but easily worsens with age, abuse in the sun, alcohol, smoking, and in my opinion, strong acid peels. So unfortunately, and you may not hear about this part, these strong peels, although exfoliating many dead cells, tend to be detrimental to the susceptible capillaries, possibly causing permanent redness.

My professional experience with glycolic peels is this: at one point in my career I worked at a salon that employed a popular glycolic product line developed by a dermatologist. We had access to different strengths of glycolic peels and were expected to perform them on our clients. Having experimented with the peels on my own skin, I found them to be less effective than the industry makes them out to be. I also noticed that the small amount of couperose I had on my cheeks became more prominent. The peels did smooth the surface of my skin, but at what cost? One more thing—the glycolic acid really burned!

So I was being instructed to do glycolic peels, which when requested, I did; but the results I noticed were quite disturbing. In addition to the positive exfoliating benefits that were occurring, most of my clients who received these peels had a noticeable increase in the redness or couperose in their skin. This was not good news. Subsequently, I found myself explaining these results to the clients, who all opted not to have glycolic treatments anymore. In place of the peels, I suggested consistent exfoliation with at-home products that were sold in the salon.

Strong peels create deep exfoliation. Deep exfoliation diminishes the appearance of lines and promotes youthful-looking skin. Therefore, it stands to reason deeper peels *should* make you look younger. Because of this promise, many people will seek out the strongest peels available. Stronger peels can deliver a quick fix, but this fast-track mentality never brings just the desired results. There is always a consequence. If you take care of your skin consistently and take advantage of professional facials, you can achieve in the long-term the benefits of short-term acid peels without incurring any of the potential damage.

Laser Resurfacing

What is laser resurfacing? The hot new Fountain of Youth seems to be laser resurfacing. This entails removing wrinkles using a beam of light known as a laser. (*Laser* is an acronym for "Light Amplification by Stimulated Emission of Radiation.") Usually operated by a dermatologist or plastic surgeon, this computerized carbon dioxide (CO_2) laser releases highly concentrated beams of light onto the skin, going as far down as the papillary dermis or inner skin. The laser quickly removes the outer skin layer (the epidermis), erasing lines and wrinkles with great accuracy. Water stored in the tissue is vaporized by the laser. As the doctor is going over an area, the vaporized skin is wiped away. A second pass is made directly over any deep wrinkles, followed by a healing ointment.

Laser surgery is usually performed on an outpatient basis under local anesthesia. If deep resurfacing is required, the surgeon may use general anesthesia. Initially, the skin will appear red and may even ooze as new collagen is being formed. It takes approximately two weeks to heal from the initial redness, and then six to eight weeks for the pink discoloration to fade away. Most reports say that within ten to twelve weeks the normal skin tone will return. There is minimal discomfort overall, with the first few days giving you the most difficulty.

The previous information was taken from literature that is available on this procedure. I have found, however, that clients who have had laser surgery experience side effects that are much more severe and longer lasting that the aforementioned time frame.

As with almost every procedure in this chapter, avoiding sun altogether would be wise. Anytime you alter the skin, you render it photosensitive, or sensitive to the sun. How sad to have gone in for laser resurfacing and come out with less wrinkles, only to incur mild to severe pigmentation problems that may plague you forever.

The jury is not out on this procedure as far as I'm concerned. There has not been enough research available on what happens to the skin in the long term. I like to give any new procedure or miracle product the five-year test. Within that five-year period you can get a good idea of what happens to the skin and how it ages after an invasive procedure such as laser surgery. Does the skin age normally after surgery? Is the skin so sensitive to the sun that irregular pigmentation is a constant problem? Are there any other negative side effects that would preclude having it done in the first place? Do most people wish they had left well enough alone, or are they happy with the results?

As I have previously said, I'm not one for altering what is naturally occurring in the skin. With time and care, your skin can reflect health and youth to the degree that your age dictates. You don't have to give in to the aging process and give up, but be careful what you try to change and what procedures or products you use. I certainly don't want to be a guinea pig, no matter what the media or the doctors say is good and safe to do.

Microdermabrasion

What is microdermabrasion? There is a lot written about this anti-aging procedure. It is the hot new miracle ticket. But I go back to my five-year test and caution you about this process.

There are no lasers or chemicals used in microdermabrasion. The procedure entails a small tube that sprays a jet of fine crystals (resembling sand) onto the skin's surface, which helps remove dead and damaged cells. It is said to be painless and does not require anesthesia of any kind. It's sometimes called a "lunchtime peel," meaning you can go in on your lunch break and come out without looking too red or swollen.

Microdermabrasion helps regenerate new cell growth. It is said to stimulate collagen production and increase blood supply to the skin. With repeated treatments, you may notice some of your fine lines and wrinkles have diminished. Pigmentation irregularities, such as hyper-pigmentation or chloasma, are said to show signs of improvement. (Remember, as long as you are prone to chloasma, it will continue to appear no matter what. This means that even if you have erased the dark spots with this or any other procedure or product, given time and sun exposure, you will be right back where you started from.)

Microdermabrasion is FDA approved and is usually performed by a licensed aesthetician. Keep in mind that not all aestheticians are skilled technicians, but everyone wants to jump on the bandwagon to make more money. Well, almost everyone—so there may be unqualified people offering microdermabrasion. I would be very careful to find someone who has gone through proper training in this procedure. Just like searching for a good aesthetician (detailed in Chapter 3), you want to ask a lot of questions and find someone who really knows what she's talking about—not just someone who wants to take your money, promising you 20-year-old skin.

Like with facials using glycolic acid, you are encouraged to get a series of microdermabrasion sessions along with using special products from the salon. Once again, if microdermabrasion is simply a mild topical exfoliation, I believe you could accomplish the same results by exfoliating more regularly at home as well as getting regular facial treatments. If you had facials as often as they have you come in for microdermabrasion treatments, surely you would see a noticeable change for the better in your skin. On the other hand, if this procedure goes deep enough to affect significant changes in your pigmentation or even your wrinkles, it scares me to think of the consequences of microdermabrasion being performed by mere aestheticians.

Although the skin is resilient, it is still a delicate organ. I don't believe in disrupting the outer dead skin with invasive or even semi-invasive procedures, but of all the current skin removal techniques, this particular one seems the most harmless. I have not seen improvements in my clients' pigmentation spots with this procedure, nor do I believe it truly stimulates collagen production. Microdermabrasion will improve the texture of your skin, as will any exfoliating process. Be aware, however, that microdermabrasion is *expensive*.

Plastic Surgery

What is plastic surgery? Plastic or cosmetic surgery is defined as an operation that reconstructs an aspect of your body into a new and different form. The term *plastic* comes from the Greek word *plastikos* meaning to mold or give form to. Cosmetic surgery is elective, nonessential surgery. These are operations you choose to undergo to correct, add to, or reduce aspects of yourself that you are dissatisfied with.

There are two main things I have to say about cosmetic surgery. First, get more than one opinion. Many books recommend getting at least *three* opinions before you let someone cut on your face (or body). Next, I highly recommend consulting a nutritionist, even if your plastic surgeon doesn't suggest you do so, to get a good vitamin and mineral program started *before* you have surgery. This will give you a better chance of recovery and possibly lessen scarring.

I have seen a lot of plastic surgery in my practice. Many clients ask who I would recommend as a good plastic surgeon. I explain it is not *only* the choice of surgeon that affects the outcome of surgery; it is first and foremost your *body* and how well it repairs itself. Do you tend to scar easily, or do you recover from wounds rapidly without noticeable scarring? Everyone's body heals differently. How healthy you are and how you heal will greatly affect how good your surgery will look.

Finding a skilled surgeon (an artist) is the second part to the "best outcome" equation. Get referrals from friends and go to several doctors before you decide on "the one." Make sure the doctors you see are members of the American Board of Plastic Surgery. This is *not to be confused* with the American Board of Cosmetic Surgery. According to Arthur W. Perry, M.D., in his book *Are You Considering Cosmetic Surgery* (listed in Suggested Reading), "The American Board of Cosmetic Surgery is a self-designated board. Its membership is open to doctors who practice cosmetic surgery but do not necessarily have the qualifications for membership in the American Board of Plastic Surgery." There are many doctors performing plastic surgery who are not members of this prestigious society. I have heard over and over again that this is the first criteria you want to look for in a doctor for cosmetic surgery.

For most procedures you will be under general anesthesia. My recommendation would be to make sure your body is in tip-top shape so you will be strong and healthy and have the best chance for optimum recovery. This area of pre-op and post-op nutrition is rarely if ever addressed. Sometimes in life you have to take matters into your own hands. In this instance, I recommend you do so. Why not go the extra mile if it could mean a better experience and recovery from surgery?

Pore Cleansing Strips

What are pore cleansing strips? Pore cleansing strips are a very well-marketed skin care fad. I wish I had been an investor in these products because I'm quite sure they have made millions. A package of six strips costs around $5. If only a fraction of the country bought just one box, well you can do the math.

When these strips first came out, every single client was asking me about them. I tried hard to find a store that had them in stock, but couldn't. Finally when I found some, I immediately went home to see what all the buzz was about. I followed the instructions, and when all was said and done, I was not impressed.

You are instructed to wet the pore cleansing strip and place it over your blackheads. (The first strips out on the market were specifically shaped for the nose. Now several companies make them for other parts of the face as well.) After the strip dries on your skin, it is ripped off (like a bandaid) to reveal debris the sticky strip has pulled out of your pores. For those of you who don't know, the main ingredient in the pore cleansing strip that does the grabbing is an essential ingredient in hair spray. It's called polyquaternium-37, and it acts like glue to pull out plugs from below the surface of your skin.

Once the strip is ripped off, the skin underneath may look red and irritated. Long-term use has the potential to cause capillary damage at the pull-off site. Yes, it does pull out some of the superficial debris that your cleanser doesn't get. Yes, it is OK to do something like this once in a while, but you wouldn't want to use these on any kind of a long-term, regular basis. A clay mask is a far superior way to deep clean your pores. (See Chapter 2/Clay Mask.) You can apply a mask to your entire face, not just small sections. And clay is soothing to the skin. Pore cleansing strips, once removed, are anything but soothing.

I'm sure these are popular with teens who think it's cool to see the junk from their pores left on the strip. Some people may see these strips as an easy way to get rid of blackheads, but be forewarned: pore cleansing strips are one of those shortcuts to good skin that do not deliver. True deep cleansing of the skin is found through consistent practice of good skin care habits, not from using a well-marketed, ineffective fad product. Like anything in life, the effort you put in usually equals the results you receive. Pore cleansing strips are a quick fix to a long-term problem (clogged pores) and will more than likely disappoint you if not cause problems with your skin. Use these strips once or twice, for novelty's sake, then go back to your more serious skin care routines.

Retin-A® (Tretinoin Acid)

What is Retin-A? Tretinoin is a synthetic derivative of vitamin A, related to a class of chemicals called retinoids. Most people are acquainted with the brand names Retin-A and Renova®, so I will use these more familiar names when talking about tretinoin.

Retin-A helps dissolve the bonds connecting your skin cells together. This increases cell turnover and can help to unplug the pores. Because of this dissolving action, Retin-A will help make the skin feel smoother as well as counteract the formation of blemishes. In contrast, in many people it also causes mild to severe irritation that leads to peeling or flaking skin. Your skin may feel smooth, but it may also look red and scaly. Retin-A is basically an irritant, and your skin responds as such.

There are still many studies being performed on the attributes or possible side effects of Retin-A, but currently some people are touting its ability to stimulate collagen production. It is also said to encourage the development of new blood vessels. As you may recall, it is the blood that feeds and nourishes the skin. If indeed Retin-A increases the amount of vessels feeding the skin, this would be a big plus. It is my experience, however, that Retin-A causes a weakening of capillaries (tiny blood vessels) in most skin that can cause couperose. This is one of Retin-A's biggest negatives.

Retin-A can help to even out pigmentation irregularities and may alter how melanin (the dark pigment in your skin) is distributed. Paradoxically, Retin-A makes your skin much more sensitive to the sun. In fact, when using Retin-A, you need to be very careful about receiving direct sunlight. Retin-A makes your skin very susceptible even to limited sun exposure.

If you ask me, all the negatives far outweigh any positives Retin-A may offer. I have seen enough adverse reactions in my clients' skin that I cannot be enticed to endorse this anti-aging miracle. Most of my clients see negligible results, if any. Because this product causes so many reactions in the majority of its users, I am amazed it is still used to fight wrinkles. Once again, the results are not long-term unless usage is continuous.

I believe Retin-A can quite often be effective for what it was originally intended to treat—acne. I am not, however, a big believer in Retin-A for helping your wrinkles disappear. Since it was developed to treat younger, acne-prone skin, most older, mature skins find it very irritating. Renova was invented to address this very problem. It is essentially Retin-A in a more emollient cream form. Supposedly Renova is more soothing and less irritating. It tends to have a lower percentage of retinoids as well.

Retin-A and Renova are dispensed by prescription only. Retin-A, in my opinion, is in the same boat with other miracles cures. Unless you have acne, I would stay away from Retin-A.

Topical Vitamin C

What is topical vitamin C? Vitamin C is a very significant vitamin. It is neither manufactured nor stored in the body, so you must get it daily from food or from supplements. Vitamin C is also important to healthy skin. It is an antioxidant, meaning it helps to keep free radicals from invading your cells' oxygen stores. And vitamin C helps in the formation of collagen.

It sounds great to think you can apply a topical product to the skin and have it penetrate down to the inner skin or dermis, affecting the collagen fibers. But there is no evidence to show that vitamin C can penetrate down that far into the true skin. However, because topical vitamin C products are generally made with citric acid, they can help to smooth texture and decompose cells. Remember, citric acid is in the alpha hydroxy acid family. So using vitamin C topically may help with exfoliation, but it is doubtful that anything more than that will occur.

I recommend getting adequate amounts of vitamin C in your diet. I do *not* recommend the abilities of a product, in this case topical vitamin C, to work miracles where miracles are impossible. Your skin acts as a barrier, keeping foreign substances from entering your body. Keep in mind that if a cream or ointment has the ability to cause a structural change to the skin, especially in the basal layer and down into the dermis, it will be classified by the FDA as a medicine or drug, not just a cosmetic. Drugs are dispensed by prescription only.

One topical vitamin C manufacturer uses a picture of an older man in its ad campaign. He has, they say, used their product on only one side of his face for a certain amount of time. I never believe these kinds of photographs. (See Chapter 16/Myth: Before and after pictures.) I wonder if there is a controlled study of this man, exactly how he used the product, and what other possible variations could have caused changes to his face. The presumption that this photograph is an accurate depiction of how this particular product works is dangerous to say the least. This man's skin is in such bad condition, perhaps *anything* he used on his face would have caused dramatic results!

I have yet to meet a client who has had any sizable results from using a topical vitamin C product. They all agree that these products are expensive and do not deliver the expected results.

In closing, I am a steadfast believer in taking care of the skin. It is my profession, and it's what I teach my clients to do. Over the years, I have seen trends come and go; fad products become popular, then fade into the void. Throughout the marketing of new products and the public's quest for even better procedures, I have plodded along—unbending. The skin is a delicate organ, resilient as it is. Because we are looking to have beautiful skin for a lifetime, steady, proven care seems the best way to achieve this. If you look back five years to what the most popular skin care trends were, few, if any, of those procedures and products are still the rage today.

There will always be a new miracle treatment to halt the aging process as well as new diets where you can lose inches in days. I want to provide an environment and an opportunity for you to let that aspect of the world pass on by. You don't have to give in to the latest trend and give up a lot of money in the process. Even if you choose to try the latest and greatest in anti-aging miracles, hold true to your skin care maintenance program (The Basics and The Extras). Taking care of your skin on a daily basis will bring you the most consistent and long-term results. I would investigate and proceed with caution if you decide to try any of the many skin care procedures available. Trends and fads come and go, but your skin must last a lifetime.

Suggested Reading

Are You Considering Cosmetic Surgery? by Arthur W. Perry, M.D., and Robin K. Levinson.(New York: Avon Books, 1997) There are many books on plastic surgery, but this little pocket book is inexpensive and answers many questions concerning all the different cosmetic procedures.

Welcome To Your Facelift: What to Expect Before, During & After Cosmetic Surgery by Helen Bransford. (New York: Doubleday, 1997) A firsthand account (complete with photographs) from a woman who had several cosmetic procedures and wrote about her experiences.

10

All About The Sun

In this chapter, I want to talk about the sun and your skin, sun protection, imitation sun, and the facts about skin cancer. If you have already had a lot of sun exposure in your life, I encourage you to get with a dermatologist *now*. Have your whole body checked, including all moles and your skin in general. Then make it an annual practice. Most skin cancers can be cured if they are caught early. If you have questions about skin cancer and sun exposure, contact a dermatologist or your local American Cancer Society. Don't wait until it's too late.

Top 10 reasons for not wearing sunscreen:
1. It makes my skin feel greasy.
2. It burns.
3. It doesn't work.
4. I just sweat it off.
5. I *want* to get color.
6. Skin cancer doesn't run in my family.
7. I never burn, so why use it?
8. It's too much trouble.
9. I forgot to put it on.
10. Wearing sunscreen makes my face feel hot.

Top 10 reasons for not wearing a hat:
1. I get too hot.
2. I sweat more.
3. Hats mess up my hair.
4. I don't have a hat.
5. They leave a funny indentation around my forehead.
6. I don't want to wear a hat.
7. I left it at home, or in the car, or at the last place I vacationed, etc.
8. I *want* to get sun on my face.
9. Why should I wear one?
10. I don't like the way hats look.
    (True, I've said I should go into the hat designing business because other than baseball caps and visors, there aren't any other choices for exercise-friendly, skin-protecting hats.)

Since different hats provide varying degrees of sun protection, the following illustrations are provided in order to show you how the sun can get to you even if you are wearing a hat.

If you are not wearing a hat, you are getting full sun on your entire face.

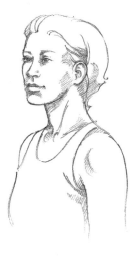

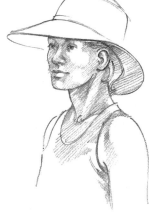

When wearing a baseball cap or visor, only your forehead, nose, and part of your cheeks are shaded.

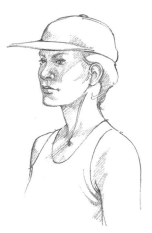

It is only while wearing a wide-brimmed hat that you are fully protecting your face from the damaging rays of the sun.

Whether driving with the top down on your convertible or with the sunroof open, you are getting a lot of direct sun exposure. In fact, depending on what you are wearing, you can get odd-looking tan lines from driving around unprotected. Bald-headed men are particularly susceptible to the harmful rays of the sun.

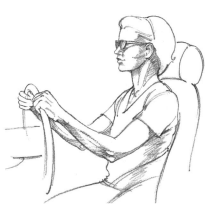

The Sun & Your Skin

The sun is the closest star to earth. There would literally be no life on our planet without the sun. There isn't anything particularly special about this medium-sized star; it shines in the same way as other stars are thought to shine. What makes the sun so important is its close proximity to earth.

The sun affects us in several ways. It has a gravitational pull on the earth's oceans, although it is probably less than half as strong as that of the moon. This affects the tides as well as the weather in general. Without the sun's energy beaming down on plants, there would be no food to eat (no photosynthesis). Sunshine or the lack of light can affect our moods. And finally, sunlight has a tremendous affect on our bodies and particularly our skin. The sun is essentially a big ball of gases, emitting all kinds of heat and energy down to us here on earth. The energy we're concerned with is ultraviolet light, or UV light.

UV spelled out. There are three basic bands of ultraviolet light: UVA, UVB, and UVC. You don't hear much about UVC light because as it hits earth's upper atmosphere, it is absorbed by the ozone layer; therefore, we are not affected by it. Not yet, anyway. With the continual destruction of the ozone layer, there is no telling what the consequences could be for the future.

UVB penetrates through the outer layer of skin, or epidermis. UVA penetrates down to the inner skin, or dermis.

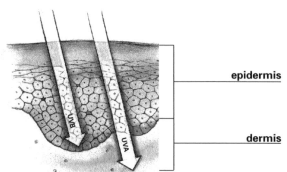

epidermis

dermis

UVB is the short ray. It hits the epidermis (outer skin) and reaches as far down as the uppermost layer of the dermis (the papillary dermis). As UVB rays penetrate the epidermis, they stimulate the production of melanin, a dark pigment that gives you a **tan**. However, UVB is predominantly known for causing **redness** and **sunburn** (UV*Burn*). It is much more intense than UVA and can cause a lot of damage to the outer skin quickly. Exposure to UVB also causes a **thickening of the top layer of skin** and accelerates the formation of **wrinkles**. In short, UVB causes **immediate damage**.

UVA is the long ray. It goes beyond the surface of the skin and is able to reach deep down into the dermis. UVA can **damage collagen and elastin fibers**, the substances that keep the skin firm and free from sagging. UVA generally does not cause sunburn like UVB rays but does play a large role in **suntans**. UVA contributes to **destroying DNA**, setting up the potential for **cancer or precancerous growths** down the road. UVA, like UVB, stimulates melanin production that can cause **pigmentation irregularities** like chloasma (hyperpigmentation). UVA causes **long-term damage**.

Skin changes. There are many reactions that are caused when sunlight hits your outer skin. Melanocytes are excited into action, which in turn produces melanin, the pigment that gives your skin its individual color or tan. Sunlight causes freckles, the color in some moles, and potentially mild to severe sunburn. Finally, DNA can be altered and may form malignancies later on.

Melanin absorbs UV light and is produced by your body in an attempt to protect itself from radiation. A tan is the body's way of responding to sun damage. When you see people walking around with a nice golden tan, they are literally exemplifying the body's magnificent response to danger. If you have a tan, you have sun damage. The two are one and the same. Black skin, however, is naturally protected (in part) from the sun due to the high amounts of melanin inherent in the skin. So if you're African-American or another dark skin type, you have not incurred damage; you are simply blessed with a built-in sunscreen from the melanin naturally (genetically) present in your skin.

A sunburn, quite simply, is caused by overexposure to the sun. It appears as inflammation followed by swelling of the outer, epidermal tissue. As the skin becomes inflamed, epidermal cells are killed prematurely. Later, this outer skin will flake off and peel. Symptoms of a sunburn include redness, swelling, and pain upon touching the effected areas. Usually these symptoms manifest anywhere from 1 to 24 hours after overexposure. Depending on its severity, the sunburn will fade after several days, leaving behind skin that is sometimes tan and quite often peeling. The type of sunburn you most likely receive from sun exposure is classified as a first-degree burn. If blisters are associated with severe swelling, it is a second-degree burn.

Sun exposure causes *cumulative* damage. This is what a lot of people just don't understand. You start accumulating "sun-time" from birth, whenever and however long you are exposed to the sun's rays. This includes walking to and from your car as well as basking in the sun at the beach. The sun doesn't differentiate one kind of exposure from the other. All exposure counts in terms of sun-time. Skin cancers can take many years to form under the surface. If you were sunbathing at 18 years old, it may take 10 to 20 years for that damage to show up.

I have sent many clients to the dermatologist to have a mole or a funny-looking spot checked out. I am noticing more and more odd places on people's skin each year. The rate at which I send people to get their skin looked at seems to be accelerating. Maybe only one in 20 clients comes back with a diagnosis of skin cancer or a precancerous growth, but I'd rather be safe than sorry. If you get facials, hopefully your aesthetician is keeping a watchful eye out for your skin, your moles (new or existing), and any changes that may occur.

Face, neck, and hands. I want to turn your attention to a few specific areas on your body where sun exposure is continual. These areas are the face, neck, and hands. They are usually exposed to sunlight all year round, especially if you live in a continually warm climate. In cold weather climates, your body is protected with clothing in the winter and therefore is safe from the sun. But unless your face, neck, and hands are constantly covered up, these areas will still be exposed to UV rays no matter what the climate or time of year.

Although exposing any part of your body to too much UV light is not desirable, it is the face, neck, and hands I am most concerned with. Remember, sun damage is cumulative from birth. Because your face, neck, and hands are exposed throughout the year (much more so than your body), this tissue is going to show the ravages of sunlight much more quickly than the skin on your body. The early signs of overexposure include lines and wrinkles, causing the skin to age prematurely; pigmentation spots, sometimes called liver, age, or sun spots; and flaccid tissue, skin that is sagging or has lost its firmness. It is important, therefore, to keep the face, neck, and hands protected throughout the year, minimizing their exposure to the sun. Obstruction (including clothing, hats, and gloves) is best for keeping direct sunlight off the skin, and wearing sunscreen on these areas helps to filter the damaging rays of the sun.

Avoid the sun? One misconception I want to address is the notion that we should avoid the sun all together. True, we don't want to ever overexpose ourselves to the harmful effects of ultraviolet radiation, but humans require sunlight in order to thrive, grow, and feel nourished. We would not exist without sunlight (as evidenced by history). The sun heats our planet and makes things grow. It stimulates certain vitamins (namely vitamin D) in our bodies and generally makes us feel good. There are studies showing that people who live in areas with little sunshine at certain times of the year have a higher incidence of depression. There is even a name for this depressed state; it is called seasonal affective disorder (SAD). We are meant to be outside. It's overexposure and unprotected sun exposure that should always be avoided, but not sunshine all together. There's nothing like a bright, sunshiny day to lift our spirits and motivate us.

Many people are sun worshipers. Their faces show the effects of long-term excessive sun exposure. Unfortunately, it seems that for every delight there is also an inevitable detriment. If you love to be out in the sun, at least one of the prices you'll have to pay will be wrinkles, not to mention the potential for skin cancer. This is especially true if your sun exposure is unprotected exposure—a potentially deadly sin.

Genetics, as with all things, play a big part in how sunlight will affect you as an individual. I know several clients who were lifeguards as teenagers and have been sun worshipers ever since, yet somehow they haven't had to pay the price (as of yet, anyway). Their skin has not prematurely aged, and they show no signs of cancer or any precancerous growths. Warning: these few individuals are *exceptions!* Genetically they have some kind of miraculous sun-protecting genes that have allowed them to avoid the damage caused by excessive sun exposure.

Most of us are not so lucky. If you were one of those kids who was out by the pool putting baby oil all over your body while lemon juice soaked in your hair, take heart. You are in the majority. Back in the '60s, '70s, and even the '80s, suntanning was the cool thing to do. Evidence of this attitude can be found in several books published up until the mid-'80s on how to get a golden tan. There was still an attitude of acceptance about getting a deep, dark tan, but in the very next decade we found out how painfully wrong we were to indulge in this activity. It's a matter of "When you know better, you do better."

Unfortunately, that saying is not true for everybody. A lot of people, especially teens, still believe a tan is cool. You'd think with all the information available to the public, people would realize the dangers of tanning and take precautions to ensure their safety and health. But we were all teenagers once, and that is not how *we* were, and it's not how teens are today. And actually a lot of adults can be found at the beach, lying out by the pool, and in tanning beds across the country. I'd like to think that when we do find out what is better for our health, we incorporate that knowledge into our daily lives, but this is not always the case. The old saying that you can lead a horse to water but you can't make it drink is still true today.

Sun Protection

There are many ways to protect yourself from the sun. It is direct light that you want to avoid in order to truly save your skin. By the term *direct light*, I mean allowing the sun's light directly onto your skin. Anytime you see the sun on your face or any part of your body, these areas are receiving direct light. A barrier is what you're looking for to obstruct the sun. The most obvious barrier would be four walls and a ceiling. In other words, being indoors. But when you're outdoors, use sunscreen, hats, clothing, and shelter such as umbrellas or shaded areas to keep the direct light off your skin.

One thing you want to keep in mind about sunscreens is that they are only protecting you against sunburn. Yes, they do filter the damaging UVA and UVB rays if you're using a full spectrum sunscreen (discussed a bit later), but filtering and totally blocking out the sun's light are two different things. Don't feel falsely armed against sun damage just because you're wearing sunscreen. But, *do* wear it. It is helpful to the degree a man-made chemical cream can be.

The bottom line: sunscreens are not a cure-all. The only true, 100% protection from the harmful rays of the sun is found inside a building, away from a window—four walls and a ceiling. Anything short of that, and you are still being exposed to UV rays. It's all a matter of preference. And if your preference is being outside a lot of the time (or even a little), you'll want to take all necessary precautions to help keep your skin as healthy as it can be—for a lifetime.

It's really just a compromise. If you're an outdoors person (like me), you will get exposed to the sun, which equals sun damage. There's no way around that. The payoff is you get to do what you love: be outside. Smart outdoors people arm themselves with all the protection they can (sunscreens, hats, protective clothing) and proceed to enjoy life. The compromise is enjoyment of the great outdoors and all the activities done outside, coupled with the inevitable sun exposure and subsequent long-term damage.

Another possible scenario is people who prefer to forgo outside activities for skin that is not damaged by the sun. These people will almost always age better (age *less*) than the outdoors type. They may not feel the need to be outside, or it may not give them the same exhilaration it does others. In the long run, they too have found what works for them—staying indoors and enjoying ageless skin. Perhaps some of these people have been fated with skin that doesn't tan but burns with limited exposure. To me, this is truly a blessing in disguise. It keeps them out of the sun and therefore minimizes sun damage and premature aging.

Please know that regardless of what lifestyle you choose to lead, sunlight can get to you when you're least expecting it. When it's cloudy or overcast, UV rays still get past the clouds and onto your skin. If you think about it, clouds are essentially water (water droplets and ice crystals). Sun rays, predominately UVA, have no problem getting through. The only time you don't have to worry about UV rays is when it's pouring down rain, because you'll be inside anyway. The sun is always beaming down UV light, even if it's a cloudy day. Sand, cement, and especially water all reflect light from the sun. So even if you're under an umbrella at the beach or by the pool, you're still getting some sunlight. Finally, it is estimated that sun rays can go *at least* three feet under water. Don't think because you're in water that you are escaping sun damage. If you are outside, no matter what you're doing, you are probably getting sun.

What is sunscreen? Sunscreen is a topical cream that contains ingredients that either absorb or reflect UV light coming from the sun. Octyl methoxycinnamate, for instance, is a chemical contained in some sunscreens that attracts or absorbs UV rays. Zinc oxide and titanium dioxide are found in many creams and reflect sunlight away from the skin. Either way, sunscreens can be effective in helping to keep your skin from burning. If you are in the sun for any length of time, however, the effectiveness of a sun product (even if it has a high SPF) will be diminished. Why? Creams are no match for the power of the sun. Remember, SPF refers to burn time, not freedom from all sun damage. I'll discuss this further later on.

Sunblock, by the way, is essentially the same thing as sunscreen, but it sounds like it totally blocks out the sun. Doesn't it? It doesn't! It's just another name for the same thing. Sunscreens and sunblocks are both helping to protect your skin when out in the sun, but both are only *filtering* UV rays. Both are keeping your skin from *burning*. So although a cream says it's a sunblock, nothing totally blocks the sun except being inside.

I have already used this example in the chapter on pregnancy and skin, but I want to include it again for emphasis. If given a choice between wearing sunscreen on my face without a hat or a hat with no sunscreen, I would *always* choose wearing a hat with no sunscreen. UV rays can penetrate through glass, clouds, and water. Why wouldn't they be able to cut right through a thin layer of cream on the skin? Obviously the optimum defense would be to wear both a hat and sunscreen, but I think you get the picture.

What does waterproof mean? Waterproof means the product will not come off in water. In other words, it's not water-soluble. It will continue to remain on the skin even after sweating, taking a dip in the pool, or jumping in the ocean. I believe anyone participating in any outdoor activities should wear waterproof sunscreen. Anything else will quickly and easily come off at the first sign of sweating or immersion in water.

What's the difference between waterproof and water-resistant? The difference between the two is basically this: a waterproof product must maintain its SPF rating (SPF 15, for instance) for 80 minutes in water in order to be called waterproof. A water-resistant product must maintain its rating for at least 40 minutes in water. Whichever you choose to use, if you are sweating profusely or are in and out of the water frequently, you really need to reapply your sunscreen.

What is SPF? SPF stands for *Sun Protection Factor*, or as I call it, Sunburn Protection Factor. The number on the product is telling you how much longer you can stay in the sun without burning compared to not wearing sunscreen at all. If, for example, your skin burns after two minutes in the sun without sunscreen, an SPF 15 will allow you to avoid sunburn for 30 minutes (2 minutes x SPF 15). This is not a foolproof system and is more of a guideline than anything else. I don't advise anyone to stay in the sun for very long without reapplying sunscreen.

Regarding sunscreens and SPFs, I have many clients who come in and say with surprise, "I wore a sunscreen yesterday and still got a tan." Unless you are wearing what would amount to a suit of armor, if your skin is exposed to the sun, you *will* get sun. Anytime you're in direct light, you will probably get some color. I wish I could tell you sunscreen is enough, but it's not. However, while it may not be total protection, sunscreen is protection nonetheless.

In Australia, they are very sun-conscious. Because the ozone layer in that part of the world has holes in it, the sun's rays (especially UVB, the burning ray) are a huge concern. I have read that manufacturers of sunscreen products are not allowed to advertise SPFs higher than 15. The reasoning is higher SPFs suggest greater protection, and the government doesn't want to confuse the consumer into thinking that SPFs higher than 15 are really arming them against extended exposure. This philosophy is not followed in other parts of the world. There is a tendency to think SPF 40 makes the skin impervious to the harmful effects of the sun.

When the SPF gets higher and higher, so do the concentrations of sunscreen chemicals. The higher the percentage of chemicals in a given product, the greater the chances for allergic reactions and intolerances to the product. Not only can really high SPFs potentially cause skin reactions, they can also make you feel invincible in the sun. The truth is sunscreen needs to be reapplied regardless of the SPF rating. Sunscreen is not a panacea for skin protection. It's just not as simple as that.

Why wear sunscreen? Since sun exposure is cumulative, you want to limit the amount of sun damage you incur over your lifetime. Sunscreen is one important way to do this. It helps to absorb or reflect damaging rays from the sun, allowing you to stay outside longer without burning. Sunscreen, because it does help filter out sun rays, can help to postpone the threat of skin cancer. Sunscreen does not prevent cancer, but it can help your skin defend itself from the harmful rays of the sun.

Sun exposure increases the already dark color of hyperpigmentation. Any amount of sunlight will do this. Just innocently walking to and from your car every day can darken these spots. If you are prone to hyperpigmentation, wearing sunscreen all the time is vitally important. Otherwise these dark, sometimes large pigmentation spots can take over your face. (See Chapter 6/Chloasma.)

What about dark skin? There are certain characteristics to dark skin that keep it from receiving severe sun damage. *However*, if you have dark skin, you'll want to heed the same warnings as those with lighter skin.

Dark brown or black skin genetically produces large amounts of melanin, giving you a dark skin tone. Because melanin is produced to protect the body from UV radiation, it makes sense that descendants of people from areas near the equator will have darker skin. Genetically you are blessed with nature's own sunblock.

It's also true that dark skin tends to age better than lighter skin because of this extra melanin production. But it is *not* true that dark-skinned people don't need to use the same common sense protection from the sun as explained throughout this chapter. If you have dark skin, please don't think you will escape the ravages of the sun. You are perhaps even *more* susceptible than lighter-skinned people. Why? Because you feel armed against the sun due to your skin tone. Therefore you may forgo wearing sunscreen and a hat. Dark skin is better protected than light skin, but you are in no way fully protected from sun damage. No one really escapes damage from the sun. Dark, light, black, white, young, or old—everyone needs to wear sun protection.

Which sunscreen should I use? This is a tough one. Obviously you want to find a sunscreen that doesn't make your skin look or feel greasy. And one that doesn't cause any irritation like burning or itching. You want to get a sunscreen that is termed *full spectrum*, which means it protects against both UVA *and* UVB rays. Most newer sunscreens on the market have both UV filters in them. Without protecting you from both kinds of UV rays, a sunscreen is only doing half its job. If you're going to be exercising outside, use a waterproof product. If you're only going to get incidental sun (like to and from your car), a regular, non-waterproof sunscreen will usually be enough.

I subscribe to a philosophy similar to the one from Australia mentioned previously. Wearing really high SPFs gives you a false sense of security. I use a waterproof SPF 25 for sports, and an SPF 15 for everyday use. I'd rather you first concentrate on always wearing sun protection and then focus on the SPF. Make sure your sunscreen (with a high SPF or not) isn't irritating or otherwise causing problems with your skin. Wear it and know that you're doing something good for your skin for the long *and* the short run.

Which sunscreen ingredients should I avoid? PABA (para-aminobenzoic acid) is widely known to be a skin irritant and is rarely used in sunscreen preparations. But it can still be found in some sunscreens, so check the label before you purchase any products. PABA "esters" are commonly used today and are said to not cause irritation. These esters are usually ingredients in PABA-free products.

Sunscreens can be tricky, and if you have sensitive skin, you may have to go through some trial and error before you find one that your skin tolerates. Not only can they cause itching and burning, but some creams may have a particular consistency or aroma that may not be pleasing to you. Any effort you put into finding a good sunscreen will pay off in the long run because you will be able to apply your sunscreen of choice whenever you'll be exposed.

How do I use sunscreen? Sunscreen can be used in several different ways. For everyday use, either find a suitable moisturizer for your skin type with SPF already in it, or mix sunscreen in with your moisturizer. Most companies don't recommend this mixing practice, but in my experience there is no harm in combining two different creams. Unless you discover a skin reaction when blending creams, go right ahead. And surely mixing a sunscreen and a moisturizer from the same product line should have no ill effects. If you are going to be in the sun for an extended period of time, you'll want to apply your sunscreen undiluted (not mixed with a moisturizer).

Apply the sunscreen to your face and neck as you do your moisturizer. If you are going to be outside, don't forget the back of your neck and ears—especially the tops of the ears. Baseball caps and visors do nothing to protect your ears. So unless you're wearing a wide-brimmed hat, your ears will be exposed. And if other parts of your body are going to be exposed, cover them with sunscreen as well. (See Chapter 12.) For daily protection of your face, however, just apply sunscreen as you would your day cream.

Sunburn Preparedness Kit

If you are going on any kind of outing, take the following items to ensure you won't have an attack of "lobster skin." All of the suggested articles will fit in a small backpack or beach bag. Don't leave home without them, or you may come back home sporting a sunburn.

Always have a lightweight, **long-sleeved, white T-shirt** (like the kind you get for running a race). It will cover most of your upper body and save you from burning. You can pull it on and off if you are boating, on the beach, or even taking a long walk or hike. It can be wrapped around your waist when you aren't wearing it. Lighter colors reflect light and won't make you feel as hot as darker colors.

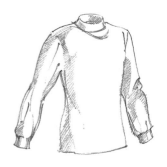

A **bandana** or **scarf** is another important sun protector. The T-shirt won't cover the nape of your neck. If you have short hair or your hair is pulled up off your neck, this area is highly susceptible to sunburn. The bandana

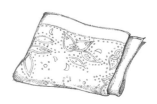

or scarf can be tied loosely around your neck, like a scout, covering most of the back of your neck. You can also dip the bandana in water before putting it on. (The water will help to keep you cool.)

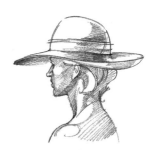

Take a **hat**. You should always have a hat with you, even if it's just a visor or baseball cap, if you are going to be out in the sun. Wide-brimmed hats offer you much better sun protection than caps, but any kind of hat is better than no hat at all. (See illustrations on sun exposure and hats on page 153.)

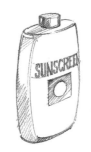

Of course, you want your trusty **sunscreen**. Waterproof is best if you are going to be in, on, or by the water. Waterproof sun protection also needs to be worn if you are going to be outside in the heat for any length of time where you'll be sweating (even mowing the lawn or gardening). And finally, if you will be exercising, then of course you'll want to wear waterproof sunscreen. Otherwise, in the first few minutes of sweating, you will be left unprotected.

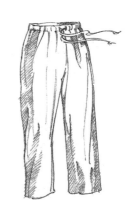

Cotton, drawstring or other **loose-fitting pants** in a light, sun-reflecting color are good to have around—especially on a boat. If your legs have been exposed for a while, slip these pants on and keep the sun away until you're ready for more.

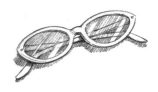

Don't forget your **sunglasses**. Most sunglasses sold today have UV sun protectors built into the glass. Check to make sure, and then make sure to wear them. Not only can they filter harmful rays from your eyes, but they will also keep you from squinting. (Squinting will rapidly increase the lines around your eyes.)

The burn. So now you've done it. Your friends are calling you "the lobster" because you fried yourself in the sun. While they're chuckling at you, you are really in pain. It's like lying on a stove top with the burners on. You're a piece of toast that stayed a bit too long in the toaster. You're overdone.

Sunburn can bring with it some serious side effects. Because you have just damaged a large section of skin, your body has been signaled to flood the area with fluids to help begin the repairing process. This will cause slight to acute swelling, or edema. It will make your skin feel tight and even more painful as the fluids stretch out your burned and sensitive skin. I want to emphasize the importance of the following advice. It has saved me and many clients from a lot of pain. I hope you never get burned, but if it happens I hope the following information can help.

If you have been overexposed (AT ALL) to the sun, start putting **aloe vera gel** all over the effected area *immediately* and *continually*. Aloe vera is 99% water, 1% protein. The water helps to replace the fluids that have been lost through sun exposure; the protein helps to rebuild damaged tissue. Aloe is a contact healer, meaning it starts to heal on contact. In cases of severe burns, aloe vera will not be enough, and you will want to seek medical treatment. But for the average, milder type of sunburn, aloe vera gel can do wonders. Don't wait until you've become a lobster before getting this product at the store, and don't forget to take it with you on vacations. Even hiking in the cool mountains can cause sunburn if your skin is overexposed.

Aloe vera products and pure 100% gel can usually be found at most health food stores. There are gels on the market with ingredients like allantoin (a soothing agent extracted from the herb comfrey) and cucumber extract. These ingredients are both beneficial in calming sunburned skin. Aloe vera gel is not terribly expensive, and it keeps for an eternity if refrigerated. It has many uses, but it is especially good for sunburns. I recommend a gel that is at least 95% aloe vera. Anything less will have too many other ingredients in it you don't want.

If you are burned, you'll need to start applying aloe immediately and frequently. Because it's a gel, it will dry fairly quickly, and you will probably go through quite a bit of it. As soon as it dries, I would reapply it. Or at least reapply it every 15 to 20 minutes for the first few hours and every hour after that for the first 24 hours. I have recommended this course of action to many clients over the years as well as using it for my own overexposure, and if you keep applying aloe gel, it can have a remarkable effect on a sunburn. For more information on aloe vera, see Chapter 14.

Drinking **water** is also important because it helps to rehydrate your system after sun exposure. A bowl of water sitting in the hot sun will evaporate in a short time. Your body, through sweating and evaporation, also loses a lot of water when out in the sun. These fluids need to be replaced often. Keep in mind, alcohol is a diuretic and leaches water out of your body. If you're drinking alcohol and are exposed to the sun, you really need to seek out some shade and keep your system hydrated with lots and lots of water.

All of these items that comprise your Sunburn Preparedness Kit (a long-sleeved T-shirt, a bandana, a hat, sunscreen, loose-fitting pants, sunglasses, aloe vera gel, and water) can easily be carried with you whenever you're going to engage in outdoor activities. Be prepared, be careful, and most of all enjoy your (protected) self.

Imitation Sun

Costly UV. Tanning beds, or as I call them, "cancer beds," are like a microwave is to a conventional oven in terms of sunlight. They emit accelerated and irregular UV radiation, amounting to abnormal UV exposure. The sun puts out ultraviolet light in a particular intensity and proportion. Tanning beds rearrange how these light rays are being emitted. And who really knows what the effects are on the human body? Do you want to be a guinea pig in an experiment involving ultraviolet radiation?

Many people are using tanning beds thinking they are safe. Unknowing tanning salon members are usually told the beds don't emit UVB radiation, and that their skin won't burn and they can tan "safely" without any worries. *Wrong!* Although people who use a tanning bed will be getting less UVB than if they were in the sun, they are still receiving *more* UVA (2 to 3 times more) than from natural sunlight. While UVA doesn't cause as many exterior signs of damage, it does cause tremendous damage you cannot see. As you learned earlier, UVA causes long-term damage, such as premature aging through damaging collagen and elastin fibers. UVA can also damage DNA, causing possible skin cancer risks in the future.

Another negative to predominantly UVA exposure is you have virtually no warning signs of overexposure. Personally, I think *any* exposure to the radiation from a tanning bed is too much. When overexposed to UVB, your skin will turn pink, then burn and feel painful. You won't have these warning signs with overexposure to UVA. Later in life you may notice a rapid increase in lines and wrinkles along with overly flaccid (loose) skin. You may have cancerous or precancerous lesions making their presence known. But by then, of course, it's too late to undo the damage done from time spent in a tanning salon. So keep in mind that when you get this kind of unnatural UV exposure, you will essentially have no warning signal if you've received too much radiation. Unfortunately, some people feel impervious to these consequences. Even though they know tanning beds are bad for them, they continue to use them anyway—even if it's just once in a while—truly throwing caution to the wind.

Fortunately, more and more information is being accumulated about the dangerous effects of this unnatural type of UV exposure. I have yet to read an article on tanning beds that gives them the stamp of approval. The only place you can find encouragement to use these radiation beds is in the brochures handed out by the tanning salons themselves. Don't be fooled; these beds are dangerous—in the short-term and definitely in the irreversibly damaging long run.

Artificial tanning. Another kind of artificial sun is achieved through the use of self-tanning creams. These are very prevalent on the market, so there are many products to choose from. They are a much better alternative than tanning beds or even natural sun exposure. Sunless tanning is a safe way to look like you have a tan without incurring any of the damage of a real tan or a tanning bed's tan. When using self-tanning products, you'll want to follow a few simple instructions.

Exfoliate all areas of your face and body where you will be applying the product for the best results. Most self-tanners employ an ingredient called dihydroxyacetone, which is essentially a skin dye. You want to get rid of any dead skin buildup so your tanning product will have a better chance of going on smoothly and staying on longer.

Shave your legs, ladies, before applying self-tanner. Otherwise some of the dyed skin may come off if you shave shortly afterwards.

Apply your self-tanning cream evenly as best you can. This can be a challenge because you really won't know if you have spread it evenly until much later. It goes on as a clear or white cream (or oil) and once it is absorbed into the skin, it disappears like a moisturizer. It's not until several hours later that the color begins to appear. Spread it onto small areas so you can keep track of where you've applied it and where you haven't.

Wash your hands thoroughly and immediately after application. If you ever forget this one step, I guarantee you won't forget it a second time! It's pretty embarrassing to be walking around with the palms of your hands and the skin around your nails stained brown. It's very hard to get this discoloration off your hands.

Let the tanning cream dry on your skin before getting dressed. Otherwise there is no telling what your tan will look like.

Sunless tanning usually lasts two to three days. After that, you'll need to reapply. Some people experience streaking or blotchiness. This can be the result of a poor-quality product, or the product might have been applied improperly. You may have even applied it too often over several consecutive days.

You may come across a self-tanning cream that just smells bad—like burned skin. This is unfortunate, but it does happen with some products. Obviously, don't use that particular brand again, and perhaps get a product referral from a friend who uses sunless tanning products.

There are many self-tanning products available, so you'll have a lot of options. There are sunless tanning creams, oils, and even self-tanners in a spray bottle. Whichever method you choose, don't forget to follow the steps listed above, and you can enjoy year-round color without receiving any of the sun damage of a real tan.

Facts About Skin Cancer

Reprinted by the permission of the American Cancer Society, Inc.

(800) ACS-2345

There are three major types of skin cancer:

- ***Basal cell carcinoma*** *is the most common kind of skin cancer. It is a slow-growing cancer that may be a reddish spot that tends to ooze, bleed and crust over, or a shiny, translucent pink or white bump, or a smooth red spot with an indentation in the middle. If ignored, it can burrow through layers of skin and bone and cause severe disfigurement.*

- ***Squamous cell carcinoma*** *may start as nodules, or as red patches with well-defined outlines. These typically grow on the lips, face or tips of the ears. Unlike basal cell carcinoma, squamous cell skin cancers can spread to other parts of the body.*

- ***Malignant melanoma*** *may originate in or near a mole. Melanomas are often a mixture of black or brown skin cells, with irregular borders. It is the least common but most dangerous type of skin cancer. If discovered early enough, it is completely curable.*

Non-melanoma skin cancers *(usually basal cell and squamous cell cancers), are the most common cancers of the skin. They are called non-melanoma because they come from skin cells other than melanocytes.*

Melanoma skin cancers *are less common than basal cell and squamous cell cancers but far more dangerous. It was once rare in this country but its rate is now increasing faster than all but two other cancers.*

Melanoma is a malignant (cancerous) tumor that begins in the melanocytes, the cells which produce the skin coloring or pigment known as melanin. Because most malignant melanoma cells still produce melanin, melanoma tumors are often shaded brown or black.

Melanoma most often appears on the trunk of fair-skinned men and on the lower legs of fair-skinned women, but people with other skin types and other areas of the skin are commonly affected. Having darkly pigmented skin lowers the risk but it is not a guarantee against melanoma. Darker-skinned people can develop this cancer on the palms of the hands, soles of the feet, and under the nails. Rarely, melanomas can form in parts of the body not covered by skin such as the eyes, mouth, vagina, large intestine, and other internal organs.

Melanoma, like basal cell and squamous cell cancers, is almost always curable in its early stages. However, melanoma is much more likely than basal or squamous cell cancer to metastasize or spread to other parts of the body. Although a few cases of melanoma that have spread to distant parts of the body can be cured, most cannot.

What are the key statistics about melanoma skin cancer?

- Cancer of the skin is the most common of all cancers.
- Melanoma accounts for about 4% of the skin cancer cases, but causes about 79% of skin cancer deaths.
- The number of new melanomas diagnosed in the United States is increasing. Since 1973, the rate of new melanomas diagnosed per year has doubled from 6 per 100,000 to 12 per 100,000.
- The American Cancer Society estimates that about 41,600 new melanomas will be diagnosed in the United States during 1998. About 7,300 people in the US are expected to die of melanomas during 1998.

The main risk factors of melanoma skin cancer are:

Moles: A nevus (the medical name for a mole) is a benign (not cancerous) melanocytic tumor. Moles are not usually present at birth. They begin to appear in older children and teenagers. Certain moles make it more likely that a person will develop melanoma.

One type of mole that increases the risk of melanoma is the dysplastic nevus or atypical mole. Dysplastic nevi (nevi is the plural of nevus) look a little like normal moles, but typically look a little like melanoma, as well. The moles can appear on areas that are exposed to the sun as well as areas that are usually covered, such as the buttocks and the scalp.

They are often larger than other moles. Sometimes many dysplastic nevi are found on the body.

Dysplastic nevi often run in families. People who have family members with dysplastic nevi have about a 50% chance of developing these nevi. People with one or more dysplastic nevi and with at least two close relatives with melanoma have a 50% or greater risk of developing melanoma themselves.

Another type of mole linked to melanoma is present at birth. This is the congenital melanocytic nevus, which is a type of birthmark.

The risk of developing melanoma is about 6% for those with congenital melanocytic nevi, and 6% to 10% for those with dysplastic nevi, although these risks are not exactly known. In contrast, the melanoma risk for the overall US population is about 1%.

Moles that are not dysplastic or congenital are very unlikely to turn into a melanoma. But researchers have found that people with lots of moles and those who have some large moles have an increased risk for melanoma. Melanoma risk is particularly high in people with over 5 large moles (over 5 mm or 1/5 inch).

Fair skin: The risk of melanoma is about twenty times higher for whites than for African-Americans. This is due to the protective effect of skin pigment. Whites with fair skin that freckles or burns easily are at especially high risk.

It is important to remember that darkly pigmented people can also develop melanoma, particularly on the palms of the hands, on the soles of the feet, under the nails, and inside the mouth. Rarely, melanoma can develop from internal organs.

Family history: Risk of melanoma is greater if one or more of a person's first degree relatives (mother, father, brother, sister, child) has been diagnosed with melanoma. Increased risk can be up to eight times greater than for persons without a family history.

Immune suppression: People who have been treated with medicines that suppress the immune system are also at risk of melanoma.

Excessive exposure to ultraviolet (UV) radiation: The main source of UV radiation is sunlight. Tanning lamps and booths are another source. People with excessive exposure to light from these sources have a greater risk of skin cancer. The amount of UV exposure depends on the intensity of the light, how long you are exposed, and whether your skin is protected. Spending a lot of time outdoors for work or recreation is a risk factor. Not protecting your skin with clothing and sunscreen also increases your risk. People who suffer severe, blistering sunburns are at increased risk of developing melanoma.

About 50% of all melanomas occur in people over the age of 50, with nearly 50% of all melanoma deaths occurring in white men 50 years of age and above. However, young people (ages 20-30) can also be diagnosed with melanoma.

Quick Tips
- Ladies, try using a tinted sunscreen instead of foundation.
- A suntan only offers you protection from the sun equal to an SPF of 2 or 3. That's it. So for those of you using the argument "Getting a tan is helping to protect my skin," you're not getting much protection.
- When looking for aloe vera, you may find both juice and gel. Aloe vera juice is primarily manufactured to drink; the gel is ideally what you want to use topically. If you're having a sunburn emergency, and the only thing available is aloe juice, use it as you would the gel. Given a choice, purchase aloe vera gel.

Important Reminders

- When in doubt about a mole or an odd-looking spot, have it checked by a dermatologist. In most cases, if it's caught early, skin cancer can be cured.
- Annual mole-checking exams are important if you're an outdoors person.
- Sun damage is cumulative from birth. Don't forget to protect your children (especially babies) from sun exposure.
- The face, neck, and hands are constantly exposed throughout the year. Don't forget to include these areas along with your ears and Chapter 12's Forgotten Places when applying sunscreen.
- Many cars have sunroofs. Be aware that when the sun is coming through and reaching your face and body, you are acquiring sun damage.
- Sun exposure prematurely ages skin—any amount, at any age.
- Car windows (glass) block out some UVB but *not any* UVA light. You are not protected from the sun when sitting in your car or near a window.
- Any and all exposure counts. Walking to and from your car, sunburns you got as a kid, driving around in your convertible, or driving with the sunroof open. All exposure counts no matter how you get it.
- Although each wavelength of ultraviolet light (UVA and UVB) causes its own set of reactions on top of and within the skin, they both can give you a tan and they both can cause cancer.
- When it comes to wearing and/or reapplying sunscreen, it's better to be safe than sunburned. When in doubt, REAPPLY.
- Sunscreens protect you from sunburn, but not from all sun damage.
- Be prepared. Don't get stuck without sun protection, even on an unplanned drive to the beach or walk in the park. At least keep a hat in the trunk of your car, if not your entire Sunburn Preparedness Kit.
- There is no such thing as a "healthy" tan.

11

The Body

Keeping the skin on your body soft and smooth comes from both exfoliation and moisturizing. If you exfoliate without moisturizing afterward, your skin won't feel hydrated and may look dry. If you moisturize without exfoliating, you are applying cream over a dead cell buildup, lessening the effectiveness of the cream. None of the following suggestions take much time, it's simply a matter of incorporating them into your daily routine. Once you see the results, the few extra minutes you spend taking care of your body will be time well spent.

Exfoliation

Exfoliation is the best way to rid your body of dry, flaky skin. There are many ways to accomplish this. Whether using scrubs, gloves, or a brush, exfoliating the dead, sometimes flaky skin on your body will go a long way in keeping the alligator look away.

Body scrubs. This is my favorite way to exfoliate the body. Because this product isn't used on the delicate and sensitive facial skin, you may want to get a large tub or tube of inexpensive scrub at the grocery store. Once you are wet in the shower, put some of the product in your hands and scrub-a-dub-dub over your entire body.

Use a body scrub after a long workout session, or whenever you've gotten really sweaty from being outside. If you have been outside, you'll have a mixture of sweat and sunscreen that needs to come off thoroughly.

Using a body scrub in the shower really does the trick as far as exfoliating dead cells and helping your skin to feel smooth all over. Always use scrubs, whether for your face or your body, on wet skin only.

Exfoliation gloves. These are gloves made of a rough, stretchy material that are great to use in the shower. They are better than a loofah because formfitting gloves can get to all the hard to reach areas of your body. Simply wet the gloves, put your favorite body wash on them, and gently give yourself a rubdown. Do not use the gloves on your neck and definitely not on your face. They are much too rough for these areas and may cause irritation. After you are through washing, be sure to rinse the gloves thoroughly and hang them to dry.

You can find exfoliation gloves at most stores that carry bath and body products. They make a great gift or stocking stuffer.

Dry-brush massage. Although this kind of exfoliation is a little more involved than just using a product in the shower, it is well worth it. Whenever clients come to me with really dry skin on their bodies, I recommend a dry-brush massage.

This procedure involves purchasing a natural-bristle brush. You can find them at most larger health food stores. Experiment with several brushes and choose one that feels just right on your skin. You want a brush with bristles that are stiff enough to stimulate your circulation and exfoliate dead skin cells, but not so rough that it hurts to use it. Conversely, don't choose a brush so soft you can barely feel it massaging your skin.

On *dry* skin, before you hop in the shower, take the bristle brush and go over your entire body using brisk movements. (Do not use the brush on your face and neck.) You are brushing off tiny particles of dead skin, and this needs to be done on *dry* skin. If your skin is wet, you will lose the effectiveness of the dry brush. I've always heard to brush in the direction of your heart. Whether there is a significant difference between stroking toward or away from the heart is uncertain. I wouldn't worry about the direction your brush is moving as much as concentrating on removing dead cells. It should be a sweeping motion on your skin. Once you have brushed your entire body, hop in the shower and rinse off.

You won't necessarily see dead skin actually coming off your body. Some of it will get trapped in the brush, and some particles are just too small to see. You want to clean your brush after each use by stroking your hand back and forth over the bristles to help release the dead skin inside, but do not get the brush wet. Depending on how much you use it, every so often thoroughly clean your brush to remove any debris that may have accumulated. Now you do get it wet by soaping it up with body wash, then hang it to dry (thoroughly) before using it again.

Your skin should feel invigorated and alive. Dry-brush massage literally wakes you up. It is great for stimulating your circulation, like a cup of coffee for the body. After your shower, use a good moisturizer or body oil all over. (See next section.) If done on a regular basis, dry-brush massage can help your skin look and feel smooth, making dried-out, flaky skin a thing of the past.

One note of caution: you may feel a slight irritation the first few times you brush your skin. Be gentle, not aggressive, as your skin acclimates to the stimulation of the bristles. After your skin has adapted, it will feel more invigorating and more comfortable to do a dry-brush massage.

Moisturizing

Another step in keeping dry, flaky skin from taking over your body is moisturizing. And like I mentioned with scrubs, I use inexpensive lotions on my body as well. Why? Mainly because the area I'm covering is large (compared to my face and neck), so I'll go through a lot of the product. Plus, the skin on the body is very different than that on the face, and therefore the quality of ingredients (which greatly affects the price) isn't as important. You certainly can use expensive products, but I find the less expensive brands do a good job when it comes to moisturizing the skin on your body.

The key to keeping dry skin away is to use moisturizer daily after every bath or shower. Remember, tap water is filled with high levels of chlorine; chlorine is extremely drying to the skin (and hair too). In order to combat the drying effects of this chemical, you'll want to moisturize your skin. This essential step is an easy habit to get into. Once you start remembering to use body cream or oil, your skin will get used to feeling moisturized and you won't forget to cover it with products.

Body lotions and body oils. Body lotions or creams (I use these two terms interchangeably) are the most common way to keep the skin on your entire body well hydrated. I recommend using a different type of moisturizer for different climates and seasons of the year. In the summer or if you live in a continually warm climate, moisturizing lotions or creams are best. Lotions are usually light in texture and add just enough moisture to the skin without feeling heavy.

In the winter or in cold, drier climates I recommend using body oils. They will be a lot more hydrating, and in cold or dry climates this added layer of oil will most likely be needed. You can use body oils in the summer and creams in the winter, but I find creams aren't hydrating enough in cold weather, and oils are too heavy in hot weather. Another suggestion is to combine a lotion or cream with an oil and smooth this mixture all over your body. If one alone doesn't feel right, experiment and come up with what works best for you.

Sometimes you're told to apply body products on semi-wet skin. The theory is that lotion will lock in any water left on the surface of your skin. However, I find this technique thins out the moisturizer, making it less hydrating. I prefer to towel off completely and apply cream over my dry skin. I do find using body oil on my damp skin is helpful. The oil is thick, and the water droplets help to spread the oil evenly over my skin.

Bath oils. These products are another way to help keep your skin moisturized. After soaking in a tub full of bath oil, your skin will feel very smooth and well hydrated. They are usually aromatic delights as well—more incense for your home. Simply pour some of the product in your bath water, climb in the tub, and your skin will soak up the oil. As long as they don't cause irritation due to ingredients that your skin can't tolerate, bath oils are a good way to lubricate rough, dry skin.

When using bath oils, there are a few things to keep in mind. First and most important, the oil will make the porcelain slippery, so be very careful when you're getting in and out of the tub. Then when the water drains out, since some of the oil will be left behind, wipe off any existing oil so an accident doesn't occur. Also, any leftover oil will cause an oily bathtub ring. Because oil floats on the surface of water, you'll need to splash the parts of your body that aren't submerged in the bath water. This will ensure that your entire body receives the benefits of the hydrating oil.

Humidifiers. As mentioned in Chapter 4/Quick Tips, a humidifier helps keep dehydrated and dry skin away. Sleeping with a humidifier lets water vapor permeate the air for as long as you are sleeping. It's a painless way to get moisture in the air, which will have a positive effect on your skin—all over.

Quick Tips

- If you don't have any bath oil, you can use a body oil in the tub instead. Just pour a small amount into the bath (a little goes a long way), hop in, and soak it up. You can also use baby oil or even an oil from your kitchen.

12

The Forgotten Places

When caring for The Forgotten Places, there are three main things you'll want to keep in mind. They apply to your body as a whole, but in this chapter you'll be concentrating on those places you tend to forget. These three steps include using sunscreen, exfoliating on a regular basis, and using a moisturizer or hydrating cream. If you start caring for The Forgotten Places now by incorporating these three steps, you can enjoy healthy, well cared for skin all over.

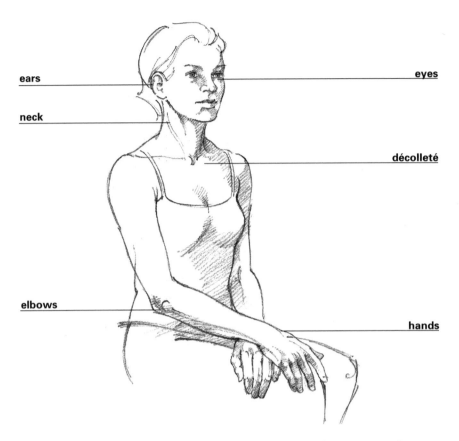

ears — eyes

neck

décolleté

elbows

hands

Sunscreen. One reason these places look forgotten is because they receive quite a bit of sun. Sun damage brings with it loose, sagging skin along with pigmentation spots (also called age, sun, and liver spots), and the potential for cancer. Start now (it's never too late) and remember to include The Forgotten Places when you're applying sunscreen to your face and body.

Exfoliation. Because exfoliation is so essential to the overall health of your skin, it is important to exfoliate thoroughly and often in most of The Forgotten Places. Getting rid of the dead skin buildup will enliven your skin, making it feel smoother and look healthier.

Hydration. Finally, extra care needs to be given to The Forgotten Places to ensure they get adequate hydration, day in and day out. Keeping the skin well moisturized makes it feel soft and supple, keeping dry and flaky skin away.

The Neck

Even though you are taking good care of your face, you may be neglecting your neck. So if you aren't already, you'll want to start including your neck in everything you do. That means your Basic 1-2-3 plus exfoliation and sunscreen. A clay mask isn't necessary unless you have a lot of breakout on your neck.

Keep in mind that when you're driving, your neck can receive a lot of sun exposure. The visors in most cars don't have any kind of extension to shield the driver's side (or passenger's) from the sun. As mentioned in Chapter 10, glass may help prevent some UVB sunlight from penetrating, but not UVA. There isn't a whole lot you can do except try to avoid long periods of exposure. If you're driving long distances, try wrapping a scarf around your neck to protect it from getting too much sun. Consider keeping a light cloth or towel in your car to drape over your shoulder and arm closest to the window. This can help keep your skin from burning while driving for extended periods of time.

The Décolleté

The décolleté is the area below the neck and above the breasts. Most women don't consider taking care of this area until it is already damaged. Low-cut dresses show the décolleté. Bikinis expose the décolleté. And rarely, if ever, do we consider exfoliating, hydrating, or using sunscreen on this area.

Because gravity pulls the breasts down (to the ground, unfortunately), the skin of the décolleté is also pulled down with age and time. In addition to this stretching, I also see a lot of sun damage on this area, which causes tissue to become flaccid and sag. Sun can also cause damage to the capillaries and blood vessels. What you might have after years of overexposure is a décolleté that is permanently freckled and brown with a slightly leathered look and a lot of broken capillaries. In other words, it has been damaged by the sun.

Start by exfoliating your décolleté. It will help to reflect the healthy skin hidden underneath, eliminating dead cells that are rarely actively removed. After your bath or shower, be sure to get body lotion on your décolleté. There is no need to use the more expensive face and neck creams on this large area, but don't forget to rub some body cream there. And don't forget sunscreen. Apply and reapply if you're going to be playing out in the sun. Even if you're not in a bathing suit but have a low-cut top or opened-up shirt, put sunscreen on your exposed décolleté. Keep in mind that even wide-brimmed hats don't shade the décolleté. So unless this area is covered up with clothing, it is constantly exposed to the sun. Try to become aware of how much sun this and other Forgotten Places are receiving. You might be surprised.

The Hands

This is another area we tend to worry about long after the damage has occurred. If you're young, start now to take care of your hands, so they will reflect this care when you are older. And even if you are older and haven't taken very good care of this area, it's never too late to start. Your skin will always reflect the care you give it. Here are a few suggestions.

First, whenever you exfoliate your face and neck, exfoliate the tops of your hands. It's a small area, so it doesn't take much time (or product), but getting rid of the dead cells will go a long way in keeping your hands looking youthful and smooth.

Next, after you have applied moisturizer to your face and neck, smooth any excess product on your hands. If they are chronically dry, apply a special hand cream or the cream you're using on your body before you go to bed. Try to apply it as often as you can throughout the day as well.

Another suggestion is to wear gloves. They can really help to keep the tops of your hands hydrated as well as protected from the elements. I have clients who sleep with gloves on to ensure an overnight moisturizing effect. Rubber gloves are great if your hands are in water a lot or even a little. Wear them while doing dishes or any other time your hands will be immersed in water. Driving with gloves on will help keep the damaging sun off your hands. Wearing gloves in cold weather will go a long way toward protecting the tops of the hands from damage, not only from the sun, but also from the dry, cold air.

Finally, wearing sunscreen on the tops of your hands is important. When applying sunscreen to your face and/or body, don't forget the tops of your hands. (See Chapter 10/Face, neck, and hands.)

The Ears

The front and back of the ears. Cleansing around your ears (front and back) is important. It may seem silly to say, "Wash behind your ears," but debris does collect in this Forgotten Place. When I'm examining a client's skin, I always lift the earlobes and check behind the ears for congestion that may be hidden there. Many times I find a buildup of dead skin and oil that could easily be removed by simply remembering to cleanse back there on a regular basis. It doesn't take much effort, just a swab behind the ears as you're cleansing your face. More often than not I see congested pores in front of the ears too. Make sure to get the cleanser all the way over to your ears because blackheads do collect there.

Along with cleansing, you'll want to exfoliate in front and in back of your ears as well. You don't need to get aggressive, but do get some of your exfoliator in that long ridge behind your ears, in back of your earlobes, and around to the front of your ears.

The tops of the ears. Whenever you will be out in the sun for an extended period of time (exercising, golfing, gardening, walking, etc.), don't forget to put sunscreen on your ears, especially the tops. Over and over again I see clients with sun damage on their ears. If you think about it, even when you wear a baseball cap or visor, your ears are totally exposed. You don't need to glob a bunch of sunscreen on your ears, but when applying sun protection to your face, don't forget your ears.

The Eyes

Although I have written about the importance of eye creams in Chapter 1, I wanted to include the eyes again for emphasis. I really feel the eye area is a Forgotten Place when it comes to proper skin care.

Many of my clients have never used eye cream before. I must admit, up until I was 30 I hardly ever used eye cream. Then when I hit 35, I started to use it with greater frequency. And now I apply eye cream many times throughout the day. Sometimes youth is wasted on the young. It usually isn't until the lines actually make their presence known that we decide to pay attention to this Forgotten Place.

As I've said previously, you have no functioning oil glands directly under your eyes; therefore you need to use cream (sparingly) to keep that tissue soft. This will not erase wrinkles, but it will keep them from furrowing into the skin. Make your under-eyes a "remembered place."

As a visual reminder, I have eye cream everywhere. It's on my nightstand, at my writing desk, and in my bathroom. I also have some at my desk in my office as well as my gym bag. I use it all the time. Not in a thick layer, but just enough to keep that delicate, under-eye tissue soft. At any given point in the day, I'll touch the skin under my eyes to see if it feels dry. If it does, I reach for my eye cream. (I don't have far to reach!) Granted, I have easy access to all these tubes of eye cream because I sell it at my office. But consider buying more than one container of eye cream. Although the investment does cost you more initially, in the long run the cost evens out. You will go through several containers more slowly than if you had only one. Whichever method you choose, don't forget to use eye cream every day (at least twice a day).

When you apply sunscreen to your face don't bypass the under-eye area. Wearing sunglasses with UV filters will also help to curb ultraviolet light exposure. Sunglasses will keep you from squinting, lessening the potential for lines.

The Elbows

Moisturizing is the most important thing you can do to keep your elbows from looking like they just stepped off an elephant. If you have a special hand cream, smooth a little on your elbows as well. This skin needs attention and should become a part of your Forgotten Places routine. You can also exfoliate your elbows. It's not something I personally subscribe to, but exfoliation certainly helps skin, no matter where it is located.

As far as sunscreen goes, when putting it on your arms, get some on your elbows too. But for the most part, moisturizing is the main step you want to include when taking care of your forgotten elbows.

Balding Heads

This is truly a neglected and Forgotten Place. I'm not going to tell you to exfoliate and moisturize this area, gentlemen. But it is extremely important to keep the sun off the top of your head. You are literally a target for skin cancer if you don't take precautions against sun exposure. The best and most obvious protection would be a hat. But if you can't, don't, or won't wear one, applying sunscreen to your bald head would be wise. There are companies that have spray-on sunscreens, making it easy to get protection on those places where your hair might be thinning or absent. My strongest recommendation is to not fool with the sun because in the end, the sun will win.

Your skin is alive and responds to care. Any attention you give the Forgotten Places will be remembered and reflected in the healthy look and feel of these areas. With just a few short minutes per day, you can help to extend the life of these areas and enjoy healthy skin—everywhere.

13

Sugar

I have a theory about sugar. Some of you won't believe it; others will no doubt find great truth in it. I believe sugar is a major contributor to skin problems and breakout. Originally I developed this point of view from my personal experiences with sugar addiction. Then as clients would come in for facials, I saw in their skin the same kind of breakouts I was experiencing. I'd always ask the same question: "Do you eat sugar?" To my amazement, invariably the answer was yes. So with my personal discoveries and with tracking the history of many clients, I have seen how sugar can be a significant contributing factor to breakouts.

I believe some people are "skin-sensitive" to sugar, and others simply are not. I find men rarely show the signs of being sugar-sensitive, and only some women do. But the people who *are* skin-sensitive do experience mild to heavy breakout that I believe is directly linked to sugar.

Sugar is addicting—physically addicting. As with caffeine, nicotine, and alcohol, your body starts depending on its daily dose. Sugar is like a drug except sugar is legal, and it's abundant. If something tastes good, it probably has sugar in it.

Sugar seems harmless because it is so prevalent, so commonplace. How could it be bad for you if it's so readily available everywhere? It's in *everything*. Aside from the obvious cookies and candies, you can also find sugar in bread, crackers, soups, sauces, and even deli turkey! Yes, that's right. Go to your grocery store's deli counter and ask for turkey with no sugar in the ingredients. Rarely, if ever, can you accomplish this seemingly easy task.

Sugar comes in many forms and is listed by several names, sometimes in disguise. Sucrose, high fructose corn syrup, rice syrup, table sugar, dextrose, honey, brown sugar, and molasses are some of the more common names used for various forms of sugar. Become acquainted with the various names for sugar and the ways it is hidden. It is in all kinds of foods you'd never suspect, so be on the lookout.

Fructose is different. This is the kind of sugar found in the fruits you eat, and I don't count fruit as contributing to unhealthy skin. But the *juices* from fruits are another story. They are highly concentrated in sugars, so I do count juices, even fresh squeezed, as contributing factors in breakouts. Let's say you use three oranges to make yourself a glass of juice. It is doubtful you'd ever eat that many oranges in one sitting, yet you are getting all the nutrients and sugar equivalent to three oranges. That is too much sugar for your body to handle at one time. It's too concentrated, and although it tastes good, I believe this seemingly harmless glass of juice will actually contribute to your skin problems.

If you can't give up your morning glass of juice, at least mix it with water—half water, half juice. This way it won't be so concentrated and will be easier to digest. This watered-down version won't taste good the first few times you drink it, but your taste buds will get used to it. So much so that later on if you don't dilute your juice, it will probably taste too sweet.

If you have problem skin and my theory about sugar as a contributor doesn't sound believable, stop eating sugar *of any kind* and see if your skin doesn't go through a radical improvement. Don't be fooled by your casual attempt at staying away from these ill-willed foodstuffs. Sugar is physically addicting, and you will probably go through withdrawals if and when you decide to kick the habit. It isn't easy.

In order to start down the path of sugar abstinence, I instruct my clients to do one thing first: read about the ill effects of sugar. Don't even stop the habit if you aren't ready yet. In fact, eat a box of cookies while you read. Hopefully, after you finish learning about what sugar *really* does to your body, you will have second thoughts about putting the evil white stuff in your mouth. At the end of this chapter, I have listed several books about sugar and sugar addiction to help you get started. Getting sugar out of your diet will probably be a slow process. Let's go over a few points to keep in mind.

Become aware of sugar in your diet. Start reading labels. You'll soon become aware (and amazed) that sugar is in many foods and condiments you'd never suspect. Crackers, breads, and cereal almost all contain some form of sugar. Steak sauce, ketchup, spaghetti sauce—you name it, there's usually added sugar, especially in packaged, processed foods. I am not implying that everything has to be eliminated from your diet, but I want you to become aware of how you may be consuming hidden sugar in many of the foods you eat.

On a recent flight, I was served the following breakfast:

- A plate filled with wonderful fresh fruits.
- A whole grain wheat cereal that had sugar listed as the second ingredient, and corn syrup as the sixth ingredient (sugars 4 grams).
- A croissant that probably had sugar somewhere in the ingredient list.
- Raspberry preserves with sugar and corn syrup listed as the second and third ingredients.
- Nonfat strawberry yogurt. Sugar was the second ingredient, modified corn starch the fourth (sugars 19 grams).
- Low-fat milk.
- A pat of butter.

According to Louise Gittleman in her book *Get The Sugar Out*, foods containing eight grams of sugar or more per serving should only be eaten on rare occasions. If you ate all the food on this plate, you would be getting well over 25 grams of sugar. What a way to start your day! Eating like this, even a few times a week, can add up to breakouts very quickly. And this is just *one* meal. If you stayed away from the cereal, the preserves, and especially the yogurt, you would be getting mostly good sugars (fructose from the fruit and lactose from the milk).

How much sugar do you consume? Do you eat sugar daily? Weekly? Only occasionally? Once you have become aware of sugar in your diet, hopefully you will start to see the relationship between your skin problems and sugar consumption.

Try a three-day sugar fast. Try taking all of the sugar out of your diet for three days—everything. Not only will you need to avoid candy, cookies, ice cream, and all of the obvious things laden with sugar, but also sauces, juice, or breads with sugar in them. After 72 hours go back to how you were eating before—if you want to. It's your choice.

In that three-day period, depending on your normal sugar intake, you may go through some withdrawals. These can range anywhere from simple cravings to mild or severe headaches, irritability (needing that 3 p.m. "sugar rush"), or generally feeling tired. The severity of the symptoms will be indicative of your level of addiction. Your body isn't used to being denied its daily drug supply, and it will rebel.

Hold on to the commitment you've made for at least three days—no sugar. But do eat well. Fruit (not juice or dried fruit) is welcome and a good idea. Oranges, apples, kiwis, grapefruit, whatever—as long as you don't overdo it. You should eat as you normally do, but just avoid sugar. You may be surprised how many foods you regularly, casually eat contain sugar. This will be a good test.

Notice how intake or abstinence affects your skin. If you start your fast with a lot of breakout, even within a three-day period you should see some improvement. If three days go by and you have no problem staying away from sugar, go for ten days. Start out with the smaller goal and see how it goes. If you can, go on to the longer ten-day time period.

Getting off sugar is hard. Sugar is physically addicting, and kicking the habit is akin to going off a *drug*. Because sugar looks innocent enough and is so readily available, it appears to be harmless. It isn't. It is a toxin in your body. Becoming aware of hidden (as well as obvious) sugar in your diet and laying off the white stuff for three to ten days will help you see its effect on your body and hopefully your skin.

Clients ask me if I've completely eliminated sugar from my diet. The answer is "not entirely." For a few years at the very beginning of my sugar discovery I completely took sugar out my diet, give or take a few lapses. Now I will eat it on rare occasions. I don't, however, give in to all of my cravings. I know for a fact my skin breaks out anywhere from an hour afterwards to the next day after eating sugar. Usually when a craving rears its ugly head, I just say no. It's not easy, but I get stronger through exercising my will. Sometimes I give in knowing I will probably break out. If I choose to give in to a sugar craving, I follow this very important rule, and I want to recommend you do the same:

Don't eat sugar two days in a row. If I follow this rule, the addiction doesn't have a chance to set in, I get to exercise my will, and I can have sugar every now and then. This doesn't mean it's OK to eat it every other day. It means don't go on a run of eating sugar for days on end. Have some cookies one day if you haven't had sugar in a while and just want to indulge. But stop there. Otherwise you will get your system readdicted and you'll have to go through the withdrawal process all over again. Don't start another chain of events. Don't link one day of eating sugar to the next. You want to break the chain, not start one.

Another alternative is to go sugar-free Monday through Friday and allow yourself a moderate amount of sugar on the weekends. It's like a reward for being good most of the week. It is the excessive intake of any toxic substance that creates the downfall of health. I'm not a big believer in complete denial or deprivation; moderation is the key here. Allow yourself some pleasure, but keep your sugar intake in check. Remember, you control how much sugar you eat; don't let sugar control you.

If you don't crave it, don't eat it. Sometimes eating sugar is just a habit. Jars or bowls of sweets are lying around your home or office, so you constantly have visual cues to eat the sweet stuff. If this is true, it will be hard to just walk past that dish full of jelly beans or M&Ms, but you've got to give it a shot. Sometimes you have to forgo the good stuff to get to the great stuff, which in this case is clear skin. So if you aren't going crazy with a sugar craving, pass up the sweets.

Don't buy things you know you're going to eat. If you are anything like me, when it comes to the junk foods you love, you have faulty willpower. I sometimes buy a sugary food thinking, "Well, I just want it around in case I have an uncontrollable craving." And the truth is, at the moment I hold that item in my hands, I know in my soul that I will be eating it as soon as I get home. This is not to say I don't give in to my cravings from time to time. But if something is sitting around my house, and it's one of the junk foods I like, I will eat it. So my suggestion is this: don't buy foods to keep around the house you know you don't really want to eat or shouldn't eat. When that major craving comes along and you decide to give in, go out and get the sweets you crave at that moment and be done with it. Make it a one-time deal. Don't keep poor-quality foods lying around in your kitchen calling you to "come and get it."

Not buying the sweet things you like may seem like a simple concept, but just wait till you're in the grocery store eyeballing all those sweet delights. You may think to yourself, "I'll just get one (box, bag, or pint) and keep it for emergency sugar attacks." Or you may think if you buy your favorite candy you'll be able to eat "just one."

My objective is to take you to the land of awareness, and to help you realize you have the ability to affect the health of your skin. In order to do this, you need to understand the correlation between sugar and your skin problems. It is within your power to say yes or no to sugar. Now *you* can decide if you want to contribute to your breakouts or not.

Quick Tips
- If you are trying to give up sugar and you have a craving or a sweet tooth, try this: take two packets of Emergen-C (see

Chapter 14/Emergen-C) in an eight-ounce glass of water and enjoy. Chewable vitamin C tablets are another alternative.

- Keep canned pineapple (packed in natural juices, not syrup) in the fridge. Although it's a packaged food that has preservatives in it, it is a cool, refreshing thing to eat, and it's sweet. Applesauce (unsweetened, of course) is another good alternative. You can purchase applesauce in single-serving containers that are perfect to take to work.

- No gum with sugar in it. That's what I would call "stupid sugar." If you have to chew, go for sugarless gum, but know that saccharin (or whatever else is used to make it sweet) is not really any better for you.

- Sugar may not cause your skin to break out, but perhaps it gives you headaches. Whatever the difficulty sugar causes in your system, the same steps apply for helping to rid it from your diet.

Suggested Reading

Get The Sugar Out: 501 Simple Ways to Cut the Sugar Out of Any Diet by Ann Louise Gittleman (New York: Three Rivers Press, 1996). I strongly recommend this book. It's a good resource guide while you are making this change in your diet, and it includes several sugar-free recipes.

Lick The Sugar Habit by Nancy Appleton (Garden City Park, NY: Avery Publishing Group, 1997) further explains about the body's addiction to sugar and how to end the cravings.

Potatoes Not Prozac by Kathleen DesMaison (New York: Simon & Schuster, 1999). This is another good book describing the ills of sugar. It talks about sugar sensitivities and how to overcome them.

Sugar Blues by William Dufty (New York: Warner Books, 1993). This is a great introduction to the ills of sugar. Mr. Dufty tells about his own battles with the white stuff and how he won the war.

14

Special Additions

In this chapter I have included some of my favorite herbs and health aids that can help keep you well. There is a plethora of natural and herbal remedies available today as well as numerous books on the subject. The following information is not the only way to keep yourself feeling good and staying well. However, these particular remedies are the ones I favor and are the special additions I share with my clients.

The following suggestions are not intended to replace or in any way be taken as medical advice. Consult your physician before adopting these suggestions or for any condition that may require diagnosis or medical attention. If you are pregnant, check with your doctor before taking any herbs or supplements or adopting any of the recommendations in this book.

Aloe Vera

I can't say enough about this miraculous herb. I have used aloe in many different circumstances, and each time it came through with flying colors.

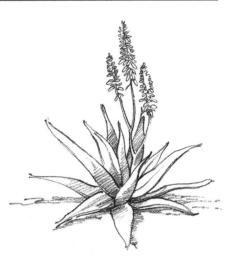

Aloe vera is my **#1 sunburn remedy**. Whenever you're going someplace where you'll be exposed to the sun, I would strongly recommend taking a bottle of aloe vera gel with you. It is easy to use and does a great job of **healing and soothing** the skin. Don't leave home without it. You can find 100% aloe vera gel at most health food stores. You don't want to use a gel that has less than 95% aloe in it. Otherwise, you may get too many unwanted ingredients along with the aloe. (I use a 96% gel with allantoin and cucumber extract—both soothing ingredients.) Simply apply the gel to sunburned areas. Because it's a gel, it will dry fairly quickly. Depending on the severity of the burn, I would apply it liberally and frequently. It works on any kind of burn, not just sunburn. Keep it on hand for vacations or whenever you know you'll get extended sun exposure. (See Chapter 10/Sunburn Preparedness Kit.)

Aloe vera gel is also good for **dehydrated skin**. If your skin has been exposed to the sun for an extended period of time (even if there is no sunburn), applying aloe gel is helpful. Because it is primarily water, aloe vera helps to replace the water lost through sun exposure, rehydrates the skin, and helps to reduce outer tissue damage.

Another way to keep general dehydration at bay on your face is to apply the gel after cleansing and before toning and using your moisturizer. The gel will act as an extra layer of hydration, adding water to the skin without adding oil. Therefore, aloe gel can help with all dehydrated skin, even if you have oily skin.

An obstinate abscess. A few years ago, my cat was spayed. She kept licking her stitches and eventually developed an abscess due to the irritation. After the vet drained the abscess, she recommended keeping the cat from cleaning the area for a few days. How was I going to do that?

Knowing the healing properties of aloe vera gel, I put it on my cat's stitches. She didn't much like the taste, so I thought it would stop her from licking the area. I kept reapplying the gel frequently, and to my amazement, within 48 hours the abscess had completely gone away, and her incision had miraculously healed. I couldn't believe it. I always knew the amazing healing job aloe could do for a sunburn, but I had never experienced its ability to heal a cut or an incision. Being termed a *contact healer*, it makes sense it would speed recovery with almost any injury.

Air bag survivor. A friend of mine called one day after her co-worker, Carol, had been involved in a car accident. The air bag deployed (which was good), but the impact had basically burned her face (which was bad). The sudden speed of something hitting your face like that is bound to cause injury. Carol looked battered and bruised, and a good deal of her facial skin was singed. I recommended applying 100% aloe vera gel liberally and frequently and told her it was to be kept on at all times. I sent some information so she'd know what aloe was and why she was using it. Then I sat back and waited, knowing aloe vera would come to the rescue.

After a few days my friend called with the results: Carol only showed a trace of the accident's effects. The burned places had healed up within the first day, and she didn't show any signs of being in an accident. My friend went on and on about how she couldn't believe the difference between seeing Carol just moments after the accident in comparison to seeing her a few days later. They were both amazed that aloe vera gel could do so much in so little time.

The following information about the attributes of aloe vera is being used with permission from the authors of *The How To Herb Book*, listed in the Suggested Reading section at the end of this chapter.

Aloe vera is one of the most popular and well-known herbs. It truly is one of the great healers. It belongs to the lili family of the succulent "aloes," not the cactus as many people believe. Aloes have been used for centuries; they have even been found in Egyptian tombs.

Aloe vera:
- *contains a pain-relieving agent and is a "contact-healer," which means it starts healing on contact.*
- *is excellent for burns.*
- *gel is used by nursing mothers for sore nipples.*
- *rapidly penetrates the three layers of skin, carrying nutrients to all layers.*
- *juice can be used as an eyedrop to improve circulation and eyesight.*
- *stimulates circulation in wounded areas, which also promotes healing.*
- *promotes removal of dead skin and stimulates the normal growth of living cells, which helps wounds to heal rapidly.*
- *prevents and draws out infection.*
- *relieves itching in chicken pox.*
- *expels pinworms. Drink juice for several days.*
- *moisturizes and improves the skin. Is put in many cosmetics and shampoos. When the product contains other natural ingredients beneficial to the skin, this is wonderful because aloe vera's penetrating ability helps to carry them through the three layers of skin. But if the products contain harmful additives, chemicals, or colorings, they could also be carried through the three layers of skin. Know what is in your product. Read the label!*

Chlorophyll

The following has been reprinted with permission from *The How To Herb Book*.

Chlorophyll is the "blood of plant life." It is the life force of plants and contains life-giving nutrients that are easily assimilated by the human body. Its molecular structure is very similar to the molecular structure of the human red blood cell—hemoglobin. It has the same effect as iron and is a natural blood builder.

Nutrition and Digestion
Chlorophyll:

- *helps to control and regulate calcium levels in the blood. Studies show menstrual blood has 40% more calcium in it than normal blood. Chlorophyll helps control this monthly loss of calcium.*
- *aids in blood sugar problems.*
- *lubricates ileocecal valve to keep it functioning properly.*
- *increases iron in milk of nursing mothers.*
- *is excellent to use in a cleansing diet because its fluids clean the structure of the cell and its important minerals build new cell life. It has been called "liquid sunshine" because it absorbs energy from the sun.*

Cleansing and Healing of Chlorophyll
Chlorophyll:

- *is a great natural healer and cleanser for chronic conditions internally and externally.*
- *stops growth and development of toxic bacteria. Disease-causing bacteria find it difficult to live in the presence of chlorophyll. Counteracts toxins.*
- *accelerates tissue cell activity and normal regrowth of cells, which helps the body heal faster.*

- *has been used in salves and ointments for external use.*
- *can be used as a gargle for tonsils.*
- *inhibits the metabolic action of carcinogens (cancer causing elements).*

Purifying Qualities of Chlorophyll
Chlorophyll:
- *helps purify the liver and eliminate drug deposits, old toxic material, chemical spray on food, artificial flavoring, colors and other coal tar products that may become stored in it.*
- *helps to get bile moving regularly.*
- *acts as a detergent in the body.*
- *has been used to remove toxic metal from children.*

Bowel
Chlorophyll:
- *deodorizes the bowel and entire body; a natural antiseptic to the intestinal tract.*
- *goes unchanged until it reaches the small intestine.*
- *aids in rebuilding damaged bowel tissue and helps to eliminate mucus.*
- *reduces acid, which produces putrefaction in bowel.*
- *helps to keep colon healthy because it destroys toxic and disease-causing bacteria.*
- *one teaspoon of concentrated chlorophyll (liquid form) to one cup of water equals a glass of green drink.*

Because the information on chlorophyll is so abundant, it is difficult to condense it. However, one thing is clear, chlorophyll is so valuable to the body that green drinks or chlorophyll should be part of a daily regime.

As you can see, chlorophyll can help in many, varied ways. It is an important addition to any **problem skin** program. When I have clients who are broken out, I ask if they are eliminating regularly, or are they **constipated**. This is important to know because when your colon is holding on to toxins (when you're constipated), many times your skin, being the largest organ of elimination, will take on the job of releasing this toxic buildup. Being broken out is a reflection of toxicity that may be due to improper elimination. Chlorophyll helps to loosen hardened debris off the walls of your colon and gets things moving along. This can help stop toxins from being reabsorbed into your body, which might otherwise result in breakouts. If you're constipated, try chlorophyll, and remember how important your colon's health is to clear and blemish-free skin. For more information see Chapter 15/Constipation.

Back to chlorophyll. One of my clients had major back surgery. She was told not to put any strain on her back muscles, including straining during elimination. Worried about the constipation she was experiencing due to the medication she was taking, my client called me looking for help. The first words out of my mouth were "Take chlorophyll." I knew it would do a lot to get things flowing and relieve her constipation. My client called back a few days later with excellent news. She was no longer constipated and therefore not endangering her back.

Chlorophyll can be purchased at your local health food store and comes in a liquid (my preference) or in capsules. Chlorophyll is basically concentrated alfalfa juice and tastes a bit like grass. Some brands add mint flavoring in an attempt to mask the taste of the alfalfa, but once chlorophyll is mixed with water, it doesn't have a strong taste. I prefer the non-mint types, but you can decide for yourself which flavor you like best. Also be aware that chlorophyll will stain like grass. Be careful not to spill it on a porous countertop or drip it on your clothes. Mixing your green drink over or in the sink would be best.

The recommendation on the bottle is to take one tablespoon of chlorophyll in a glass of water twice daily. If you have breakout, I recommend taking four tablespoons in water twice a day for at least three to four weeks. You want to get enough chlorophyll in your system to effect a change. After a month or so of using this higher dosage, you can take one tablespoon twice a day if you prefer or continue with the higher dose. Four tablespoons is equivalent to a full shot or saki glass.

Consider taking a small bottle of chlorophyll with you if you tend to get constipated while traveling. If I'm going to a city where I know I can pick some up at a health food store, I'll wait to buy it. Chlorophyll needs to be kept in glass, and because it stains, you certainly don't want the bottle to break in your travel bag. I recommend putting it in one or two Ziploc baggies just to be safe. If that's too much trouble, chlorophyll does come in capsule form.

Echinacea

Echinacea is one of the best-known herbs for stimulating the immune system. It is used to fight against **colds, flu,** and **minor infections.** The echinacea plant is a beautiful purple coneflower resembling a hot-pink sunflower and is indigenous to North America. Native Americans knew of echinacea's powerful healing abilities and often used it to treat colds, flu, and other ailments. Echinacea is

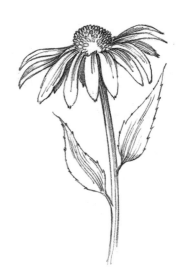

essential to have around at all times—at home, in your travel bag, and at the office.

Whenever you get sick, it's a breakdown of your immune system on some level. So taking supplements to boost it back up will help keep you healthy. Echinacea increases the activity of the immune system.

According to the Herb Research Foundation (800-748-2617), "Unlike a vaccine, which is active only against a specific disease, echinacea stimulates the *overall* activity of the cells responsible for fighting infections. Unlike antibiotics, which are directly lethal to bacteria, echinacea makes our own immune cells more efficient in attacking bacteria, viruses, and abnormal cells. Echinacea facilitates wound healing and speeds recovery from viruses."

To help keep your body's defenses strong against infection, it is important to take enough echinacea and to take it often. But also be aware that with long-term use, it appears echinacea will lose its effectiveness. Six to eight weeks seems like the maximum time period for continuous beneficial usage. Although it's not effective to take it over long periods of time, the benefits of taking echinacea for a short time are numerous. The rule of thumb I follow is to take supplements only when needed. There is no known toxicity to echinacea.

I use a product that has echinacea as well as golden seal and garlic. (Golden seal and garlic are also immune system stimulants.) Individually these herbs can work wonders; together they pack a powerful punch to fight against infections. Whatever you decide to take, I highly recommend having echinacea or echinacea and golden seal on hand for those times when you need an extra immune system boost.

Emergen-C

Whether or not you're a vitamin taker, you may want to consider taking vitamin C. It is vital to proper body function, yet it is the only vitamin that is neither manufactured nor stored in the body. This means you must get it in your diet on a daily basis either by supplements or in your food. My favorite way to get extra vitamin C (other than through fruits and vegetables) is with a 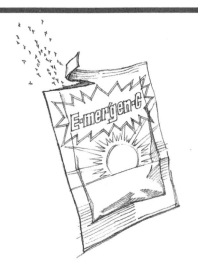 product called Emergen-C. It is a powder that comes in single-serving packets. Most larger health food stores carry it. Mix two packets in eight ounces of water once a day, several times a day, or whenever you feel you need an extra boost. If I'm fighting something off, I will take two packets every hour for at least four to five hours. Vitamin C is easily destroyed by stress, alcohol, smoking, and pollution. Whatever vitamin C your body doesn't absorb is filtered out through your urine, so there is no real threat of taking too much vitamin C.

Sugar substitute. If you're craving sweets but trying to stay away from sugar, take two packets of Emergen-C in a glass of water and enjoy. This will help to quench your desire for sweets because this vitamin drink is very sweet on its own, so you don't have to put any "bad" sugar into your system. Emergen-C is available in several flavors, and all of them taste sweet and can help to curb your sugar cravings.

Evening Primrose Oil

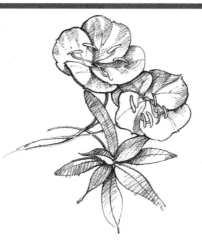

I was first introduced to evening primrose oil when I had very oily skin that was prone to breakout. The reason I started taking this supplement, however, was to help me through the intense pain I used to have with menstrual cramps. Evening primrose oil really helped to ease the tension brought on by **PMS** and helped alleviate a lot of the discomfort from **cramps**. At the same time I noticed evening primrose oil seemed to be helping with my **breakouts** and even the overall **oiliness** of my skin. I started suggesting it to my clients with problem skin, and they also had similar results.

Evening primrose oil contains high levels of essential fatty acids (EFAs). These fatty acids are necessary in the production of prostaglandins, which are hormonelike substances. These substances are vital in regulating different systems in the body, including your oil glands. Therefore, getting an adequate supply of EFAs can actually help to *reduce* oiliness.

If you decide to try evening primrose oil, you'll have to experiment with dosage to find what works for you. For PMS and cramping, I usually take 1-2 capsules morning and night at the onset of ovulation and increase the dosage to maybe 3-4 capsules twice daily until the end of my period. For problem skin, you might try 2 capsules twice daily. If you don't notice improvement, try up to 4 capsules two times a day and see if that brings about a positive change in your skin.

Evening primrose oil is also another **hangover helper**. Six to ten capsules taken before bed on a night you had (perhaps too much) alcohol will go a long way to reduce the symptoms of a hangover.

Garlic

Garlic is another herb proven to help strengthen your immune system. Traditional uses for garlic include **colds, flu** and other **infections, earaches, yeast infections**, and **high blood pressure**. Garlic reduces cholesterol levels, has a blood-thinning effect, and is said to lower blood pressure. Known as a medicinal "food," this intensely studied herb has impressive test results. Garlic is an **antimicrobial**,

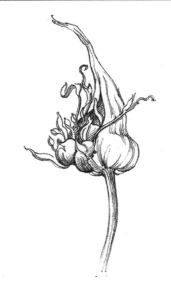

and according to the Herb Research Foundation, it was used by priests in the Middle Ages to protect themselves against bubonic plague (the powerful bacterial infection that was taking over the European countryside).

Heat (cooking) destroys the allicin in garlic. Allicin, sometimes called nature's penicillin, is the antibiotic component that kills bacteria and many viruses. So to receive the medicinal properties of garlic, it must be eaten raw (one or two cloves equal one dose), or in liquid or pill form. Eating raw garlic is a great way to infuse your system with garlic's healing properties. I love garlic, but eating it raw as a medicine isn't my cup of tea. There are several brands of garlic pills out on the market that are coated in a way so the allicin (the odor-producing component) digests in the small intestines. Broken down there, you get none (or hardly any) of the bad breath side effects, and your immune system gets all the medicinal benefits. So never fear, science has come up with a solution to the problem of garlic breath. If you choose to eat garlic raw, eat a few stems of parsley (a natural breath freshener), or put a drop of essential oil of peppermint on your tongue to help alleviate garlic breath.

I've included the following information from *The How To Herb Book*. It is reprinted with permission.

Garlic is called nature's antibiotic. It contains allicin, a natural antibiotic. One milligram of allicin has a potency of 15 standard units of penicillin. It is effective against toxic bacteria, viruses, and fungus. Garlic contains more germanium, an anticancer agent, than any other herb. In tests with mice and rats, garlic-fed groups developed no cancer—where nongarlic-fed groups developed some cancers. In Russia, garlic was found to retard tumor growth in humans.

Garlic:
- *is active against staphylococcus and E. coli bacteria.*
- *is good to take for all diseases (antibacterial, antifungal, antiviral, anticancer) including contagious diseases.*
- *protects against infection.*
- *has detoxifying effects on all the body systems.*
- *improves, tones, and strengthens the entire physical condition. Has a rejuvenating effects on all cells.*
- *builds endurance and energy.*
- *strengthens body defenses against allergens.*
- *has soft oils that help to emulsify plaque and loosen it from arterial walls.*
- *contains selenium, which helps arteriosclerosis.*
- *strengthens blood vessels.*
- *equalizes blood vessels.*
- *equalizes blood pressure, high or low.*
- *has a sugar-regulating factor.*
- *taken internally is one of the most effective herbs for killing and expelling parasites.*

- *is used in enemas. Besides being used as straight garlic enema, it is excellent to combine with catnip for a catnip/garlic enema. The catnip pulls mucus and soothes the cramping of the colon, etc. The garlic kills the germs and parasites, improves peristaltic action, and also pulls mucus.*
- *contains protein, phosphorus, potassium, vitamins A, B, B2, and C, calcium, sulfur, selenium, germanium, allicin, allicetoin I and II, aluminum, chlorine, manganese, zinc, copper, and iron.*

Lysine

If you have the herpes virus, you know how debilitating it can be. The trick to keeping the painful sores from appearing in the first place is to recognize the early warning signs and take care immediately. At the first sign of an outbreak (usually a nerve twinge or tingling at the spot your herpes manifests), (a) take your prescription medication if you have one (Zoviraz or other prescription brands), or (b) take lysine, which is an amino acid that has been found to help with the **herpes virus**. Don't wait for the sore (sometimes referred to as a cold sore) to make its presence known before you take something for it. If you act quickly, it can help prevent the long and arduous task of living with a herpes sore.

The following has been reprinted by permission from *The How To Herb Book.*

L-lysine is an enzyme that has been found to help the cold sore virus, Herpes I and II. At the first sign or start of cold sore or canker, taking one 500 mg. tablet of lysine has been effective in preventing them from occurring. (Aloe vera also contains this enzyme.) Some people who have had trouble with cold sores and cankers all their lives have started taking one lysine tablet each day and have had no more problems with them.

Excess arginine, an amino acid which is in large concentration in chocolate and nuts, is thought to be a contributing cause of cankers and cold sores. Lysine and arginine balance each other. When cankers or cold sores exist, arginine is in excess and extra lysine is needed to bring the body back in balance.

Water

Top 10 excuses for not drinking water:

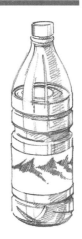

1. I don't get thirsty.
2. I don't like the way water tastes.
3. It makes me have to go to the bathroom—a lot.
4. I forget to drink it.
5. I don't sweat, so I don't need much water.
6. I've never been a water drinker, and I'm doing fine without it.
7. It makes me feel bloated.
8. When I walk around, my stomach sounds like a washing machine.
9. I don't have time to drink all the water I need to.
10. The water in my city doesn't taste good and I don't want to buy water.

What are your top 10 excuses? People have many excuses for not drinking enough water. But I hope by the end of this section you will be convinced to **drink more water!**

Water is essential to all life. But do you know why? I am including, in its entirety, a handout on the importance of water. I was unable to locate the author, Bob Hoffman, who deserves every bit of credit for this wonderful piece.

All Life Depends Upon Water
by Bob Hoffman

All life depends on water.

Breathing, digestion, elimination, glandular activities, heat dissipation, and secretion can be performed only in the presence of water solutions.

The role of water in metabolism, in assimilation, in regulating body temperatures, and in nourishing the tissues explains why we cannot survive very long without adequate amounts of water.

While the average person (128 pounds for women, 154 pounds for men) in the temperate zone may "get along" on six pints of water daily if he or she is only moderately active, two to four times as much are needed during periods of vigorous exercise or work, particularly in hot or humid weather. When I had my biggest day as an athlete, competing in 13 races in one day, finishing not worse than third in any one of them, I weighed 167 to start, 154 at the end of the day. By coincidence, I averaged a loss of a pound a race.

Almost without exception, a domestic animal, horse, cow, pig, dog or cat, will upon arising take a drink of water if it is available. The custom of early morning drinking of water should be universally followed.

Most people do not drink enough water. When taken by the glassful, a fair measure is consumed, but when drinking fountains are present, a drink is usually a small mouthful.

With every meal, about a pint of saliva, which is over 99 percent pure water, is secreted by the salivary glands of the mouth and swallowed to make possible the digesting of food.

Approximately 96 percent of one's perspiration is water, so when I lose an average of four pounds in an hour of weight training and running, I have lost mostly water, but the other four percent represents a loss of calories and fat also.

The quantity of water excreted by the kidneys is almost in direct proportion to the amount of water taken into the body. The quantity eliminated by the kidneys varies from three pints to one gallon daily, although in certain forms of physical irregularity, notably diabetes, as much as three gallons of water is eliminated in 24 hours.

Increased elimination by the kidneys will lower blood pressure. R. Lincoln Graham, M.D. who spent his life practicing hydrotherapy instead of drug therapy, stated that "...thus it is a very splendid rule in all conditions of excessive blood pressure, to drink on an empty stomach, large quantities of water, which will result in excessive stimulation of the kidneys, long after the water is eliminated. In this respect water is a remedy without a rival." When a doctor finds that the diastolic blood pressure is very high, he looks for kidney trouble.

More water in the system is a great help to elimination. When there is too little water in the system, it is taken first for necessary processes and there is not enough to materially aid elimination. The stool is hard and dry, and defective drainage, which many authorities call "the disease of disease" is the unfavorable result.

It is so much better to have too much water in the body than not enough. The kidneys will eliminate any surplus with surprising speed, but nothing but harm to the efficiency of the body will accrue when there is not enough water.

You will notice that we say drink more water. Not more sugar laden soft drinks or more coffee. Most soft drinks are strictly a chemical product. When the sugar is not used in their manufacture, only a synthetic sweetener, the manufacturers of such products advertise that the drink contains less than one calorie. This indicates that it indeed has no food value. Good water is the best answer.

The Department of Agriculture book on water states, "How far most of us have strayed from the old family spring. Generations of men and women have grown up without experiencing the joy of satisfying their thirst from cool, sparkling spring water."

You will be wise to drink more water, much more water. Too much water is not harmful, as the kidneys remove the surplus, but too little water can indeed be harmful to the body, which of course is YOU.

How Eight Glasses A Day Keep Fat Away

Incredible as it may seem, water is quite possibly the single most important catalyst in losing weight and keeping it off. Although most of us take it for granted, water may be the only true "Magic Potion" for permanent weight loss.

Water suppresses the appetite naturally and helps the body metabolize stored fat. Studies have shown that a decrease in water intake will cause fat deposits to increase, while an increase in water intake can actually reduce fat deposits.

Here's why: the kidneys cannot function properly without enough water. When they do not work to capacity, some of their load is dumped onto the liver.

One of the liver's primary functions is to metabolize stored fat into usable energy for the body. But if the liver has to do some of the kidney's work, it cannot work at full throttle. As a result, it metabolizes less fat, more fat remains stored in the body, and weight loss stops.

Drinking enough water is the best treatment for fluid retention. When the body gets less water, it perceives this as a threat to survival and begins to hold on to every drop. Water is stored in extracellular spaces (outside the cells). This shows up as swollen feet, hands, and legs. Diuretics offer a temporary solution at best. They force out stored water along with some essential nutrients. Again, the body perceives a threat and will replace the lost water at the first opportunity. Thus, the condition quickly returns. The best way to overcome the problem of water retention is to give your body what it needs—plenty of water. Only then will stored water be released.

If you have a constant problem with water retention, excess salt may be to blame. Your body will tolerate sodium only in certain concentrations. The more salt you eat, the more water your system retains to dilute it. But getting rid of unneeded salt is easy—drink water. As it is forced through the kidneys, it removes excess sodium.

The overweight person needs more water than the thin one. Larger people have larger metabolic loads. Since we know that water is the key to fat metabolism, it follows that the overweight person needs more water.

Water helps to maintain proper muscle tone by giving muscles their natural ability to contract and by preventing dehydration. It also helps to prevent the sagging skin that usually follows weight loss. Shrinking cells are buoyed by water, which plumps the skin and leaves it clear, healthy, and resilient.

Water helps rid the body of waste. In weight loss, the body has more waste to get rid of—all that metabolized fat must be shed. Again, water helps flush out waste.

Water can help relieve constipation. When the body gets too little water, it siphons what it needs from internal sources. The colon is a primary source. Result? Constipation. But when a person drinks enough water, normal bowel function returns.

So far, we have discovered some remarkable truths about water and about weight loss: the body will not function properly without enough water and cannot metabolize stored fat efficiently. Retained water shows up as excess weight. To get rid of excess water you must drink more water. Drinking water is essential to weight loss. How much water is enough? On the average a person should drink eight 8 oz. glasses every day. However, the overweight person needs one additional glass for every 25 pounds of excess weight. The amount that you drink should be increased if you exercise or if the weather is hot and dry. Water should preferably be cold—it's absorbed more quickly into the system than warm water. Some evidence suggests that drinking cold water can actually burn calories.

When the body gets the water it needs to function optimally, its fluids are perfectly balanced. When this happens, you have reached the "breakthrough point." What does this mean? Endocrine gland function improves. Fluid retention is alleviated as stored water is lost. More fat is used as fuel because the liver is free to metabolize stored fat. Natural thirst returns. There is a loss of hunger almost overnight. If you stop drinking enough water, your body fluids will be thrown out of balance again and you may experience fluid retention, unexplained weight gain and loss of thirst. To remedy this situation you have to go back and force another breakthrough.

Drinking enough water can sometimes feel like a daunting task day in and day out. Before I give you water drinking tips, I want to offer you a different way to look at water in the foods you eat. Let me illustrate this point with an example. When I asked a client of mine if she drank much water she said, "I eat a lot of fruits and vegetables." Although these foods do contain a good deal of water, it still takes water to digest them. Fruits and vegetables are high water-content foods and are fairly easy to digest but still don't count toward your eight glasses a day. Concentrates such as sugar, salt, pasta, bread, and even meats take a lot of water to digest. These foods are low in water-content, and your body requires a lot of water to assimilate and break them down. Everything *except water* requires water in order to be digested in the body. Coffee, tea, and even sodas don't count as water intake. These, too, require water to be digested. In fact, caffeine and alcohol act as diuretics and actually leach water from your body. Sodas contain water but loads of chemicals as well, so it takes a lot of water to flush these toxins out of your system. Drinking clean, filtered water is the only water that counts toward your daily intake. Remember, eight 8-ounce glasses is the minimum daily recommendation. Most people don't get enough water, so I'm including a few tips that may help to remind you to *drink more water.*

Visual stimulants or timing cues can be helpful reminders to consume water. Using drinking glasses you like will help to stimulate your reflex to drink water. Recently I purchased some great eight-ounce drinking glasses. They are short, so it seems like I don't have to drink a lot of water. It's a visual thing. I love these glasses, and I actually like going into my kitchen and grabbing one, filling it with clean, filtered water, and drinking one or two glasses. (I'm not a sipper. I drink a whole glass at a time.) I always keep an empty glass on my kitchen counter to remind me to fill it up, then I down another eight ounces of the clear stuff.

There are countless ways to get yourself to drink more water. In the morning, when you first get up, try drinking one or two glasses. It will put some water immediately into your system and hopefully get you started on a day filled with water. When you arrive at work, drink a glass, and before you leave for the day drink another one. Eleven a.m., 3 p.m.—one glass each. In just doing that, you've gotten several glasses in without much effort. On the commute to and from work, drink bottled water you keep in the car (or your bag, briefcase, backpack, etc.). Wherever and whatever works for you, find creative ways to get more water into your system. It's a constant battle, but visual stimulants and timing cues can help ensure you drink enough water every day.

Quick Tips

- Grow aloe at home. Aloe vera plants are very easy to take care of. In fact, the less care you give them, the better they seem to do. They require very little attention, just a little water here and there. After all, they grow in the desert, so they are no stranger to barren conditions. I highly recommend having one either inside or outside your home. Then you're sure to have 100% aloe gel available to you at all times. Simply break off a mature leaf and squeeze the succulent juice out onto the injured area.
- Part of the trick to not getting sick is to catch germs early. Most illnesses have early warning signs. Sometimes it's a headache, perhaps muscle aches, or just a "funny feeling." If you've been around a person with a cold or the flu, you are more susceptible

than if you hadn't had contact. Be aware of any odd sensations or feelings in your body, including thoughts like "I wonder if I'm getting sick." Then act immediately on these feelings. The longer you wait, the more time you give the germs to manifest into a cold or the flu. Act quickly and stay well.

- Take Emergen-C to work, and instead of the usual 11 a.m. or 3 p.m. cookie or cup of coffee, mix a couple of packets in a glass of water and have a refreshing health drink.
- Emergen-C is great to take on hiking or camping trips (or whenever you're traveling). You can even sprinkle small amounts of the powder on your tongue. It's tangy, which makes your mouth water, and on a long, hot trek this can feel most refreshing.
- Why put ice cubes made with tap water into a glass of clean, filtered water? Make ice cubes with filtered water too.
- Since restaurants rarely serve filtered water, always ask for a lemon wedge and squeeze the juice into your water. Lemon juice contains antibacterial and astringent properties that are good for internal cleansing.

Suggested Reading

Aloe Vera: Nature's Legendary Healer by Alasdair Barcroft (London: Souvenir Press, 1997) is a comprehensive and practical book that will guide you into the many uses of this medicinal, healing plant.

Evening Primrose Oil by Judy Graham (Rochester, Vermont: Thorsons Publishing Group, 1990) explains in great detail all the complexities of this remarkable botanical specimen in an easy-to-understand format.

The Family Herbal by Barbara and Peter Theiss (Rochester, Vermont: Healing Arts Press, 1993) is a wonderful guide to the medicinal qualities of plants and herbs. They give easy-to-use instructions for making teas and tinctures as well as other applications for your family's health care.

The How To Herb Book by Velma J. Keith and Monteen Gordon (Pleasant Grove, Utah: Mayfield Publications, 1994) is my favorite herb book of all time. This is a good reference book for all kinds of ailments, including detailed descriptions of herbs, vitamins, and minerals essential to good health. I love this book! If you can't find it in the bookstores, write to the publishers at Mayfield Publication, P.O. Box 157, Pleasant Grove, Utah 84062.

The New Natural Family Doctor: The Authoritative Self-Help Guide to Health and Natural Medicine by Dr. Andrew Stanway (Berkeley, CA: North Atlantic Books, 1996) is a well written and comprehensive self-help guide to natural medicine. It covers everything from exercise to massage, illness to natural therapies. It makes a great reference book.

15

Mixed Bag of Tips

When I work with my clients, it is never just topically or "skin deep." I try to help them on many related issues by sharing tidbits of information I may have. So this is a mixed bag of tips that may or may not directly pertain to healthy skin, but all of the following sections do affect your health in one way or another. I have added certain sections because I wanted to help you, the reader, on more than just a skin-deep level.

What To Do

Airplanes. If you are a frequent flyer, you don't need me to tell you how hard flying is on your skin. There are several things you can do to help lessen the effects of air travel, but nothing short of taking the train will completely eliminate all the symptoms you may encounter.

One way to help your skin is to exfoliate before and after your flight. This will help lessen the dead cell buildup before traveling and get rid of dehydration after your flight. If exfoliating both before and after is not possible, at least do one or the other. When I was on a long trip (Dallas to Australia), I went into the bathroom and exfoliated midflight. It really helped my skin look and feel refreshed after the long trip. You can benefit from doing this on short excursions too.

Applying a hydrating gel or mask underneath your moisturizer is another way to help curb the dehydrating effects of flying. Even applying aloe vera gel under your creams is an option. You are trying to hold as much moisture in your skin as possible, and putting gels underneath your hydrating cream can really help. Please note that if you're going to add this step, there is a particular order I recommend: cleanse, put the gel on, spray your toner, then apply your moisturizing cream. The gel and the cream will tend to stick together, making the application of your cream difficult. By putting the gel on first and then your toner, you'll have a better chance of a smooth application.

Finally, take a water mister with you on all flights. Spraying your face with water will superficially hydrate your skin, helping to replace the moisture that is lost from the dry air in an airplane.

Skiing. This is a tough one. Skiing is one of the harshest environments for the skin. Not only are you faced with sun exposure and sun reflection from the snow, but you may also encounter windburn along with cold, dry air in the mountains. I wish the ski masks that we used to wear as kids, the kind with holes for your eyes and nose, were fashionable. Because short of wearing one of these, your skin is going to be ravaged from skiing. There's no way around it.

Wearing sunscreen (waterproof with a high SPF) is an absolute must. If your ears (or any of The Forgotten Places) are going to be exposed, be sure to cover them with sunscreen. Under-moisturizer helpers such as aloe gel or a hydrating mask (discussed earlier under Airplanes) are really helpful. And keeping your face covered as much as possible is really important. I know skiing is not only a sport, but it is many times a fashion statement as well. I doubt adults are going to suddenly don the ski masks I spoke of earlier. But do be cognizant of how much sun your exposed body parts are receiving. Make sure to keep moisturizer and sunscreen on, and basically *protect your skin*. Then ski safely and have a great time swooshing down the slopes.

Cold weather. In the winter months, all the exfoliation in the world does not stop most skin from feeling dehydrated. I keep my house very warm in the winter, and therefore the artificial heat tends to dry the air out as well as my skin. I exfoliate more regularly (sometimes every day), and I also begin to add special hydration helpers (special oils or glycerin-based ampoules) to both my day and night creams. Sometimes in the dead of winter, I will also put on a hydrating gel underneath my creams to add even more moisture to my skin. A humidifier is another consideration. It will add moisture to the air and can be used in your bedroom while you sleep.

Hot weather. Drinking sufficient water in hot weather cannot be stressed enough. Dehydration—not only of the skin, but also of the body—is a serious side effect of not getting enough fluids internally. This is especially evident during hot weather. Along with water, taking Emergen-C is helpful. It replaces electrolytes and minerals as well as vitamin C, which are all easily lost due to sweating. Keep in mind, sweating is like your body's air conditioner. It helps to keep your body's temperature down. Although you may not notice profuse sweating (like during exercise), your "air conditioner" is constantly on, and you are constantly sweating to some degree. So *drink plenty of water!*

As for your skin, don't forget to exfoliate and use a clay mask. Heat activates all glandular activity, and this includes your oil glands. In the summer months, even people who normally don't have any problems with their skin may experience at least minor breakout. This can be chalked up to the heat. You're sweating more, your oil glands are working harder, and your whole body is trying to keep itself cooled down and functioning properly in the heat. It's not uncommon to have more than normal breakout during hot weather.

Stay cool, well hydrated, and keep up with your daily 1-2-3 plus The Extras program. Of course, you'll want to always be armed with sunscreen (preferably waterproof) all during the summer. You'll be outside more, in the sun more, and you'll need to apply your sunscreen more often. To refresh your memory on protecting your skin in the sun, refer back to Chapter 10.

Dry and desert climates. If you live in a desert climate, your skin will naturally be drier. The dry air will soak up a lot of the natural moisture (water) and oil from your skin. I moved to Los Angeles many years ago, and before I left Texas, my skin was oily. After living in L.A. for a year, I noticed significant changes in the oil levels of my skin. It had gone from oily to normal. Throughout the years I have heard similar stories from clients whose skin changed due to climate changes. Perhaps they lived in a desert climate, and then they moved south where it's humid. These people suddenly began to experience skin problems. And the opposite can also happen. Going from humid air to drier, desert-type locations, problem skin may clear up. (Although the dry climate may cause problems with dryness or dehydration.)

Dry air plus cold wind can really be hard on your skin. If you live in a dry climate like Colorado, you are well aware of how it affects your skin. Unfortunately, there is no miracle cure for what these environments do to the skin. Being consistent about exfoliating and using good moisturizers is imperative. Without being diligent, you will be faced with very dried-out skin. Using gels underneath your moisturizing creams can help lock in moisture that is lost through constant exposure to dry air.

One year I had two clients who moved to Denver. They left Texas with its humid, flat environment for the beauty of Colorado. It wasn't long after their moves that they called me, frantic about the dryness they were both experiencing. The air in Denver was very dry, and the water was hard. (The water in Colorado contains a high-mineral content that is drying to the skin.) I started out having them exfoliate with a gommage every day or at least two to three times per week. (Exfoliation always rescues your skin from dryness and/or dehydration.) One of these clients also had oily, problem skin. I couldn't change her moisturizer because I first needed to address her overactive oil glands. It was the surface of her skin that was dried out, not her oil glands. If she had gone to a department store, they might have started her down the road to disaster—moisturizers and other products for dry skin. Her skin wasn't dry; it was *dehydrated*. This is always an important difference to be aware of. (See Chapter 4.) Next I had her use a hydrating gel underneath her moisturizer. This added extra moisture to her skin's surface without adding extra oil. The combination of the two, exfoliation plus a hydrating gel, seemed to do the trick.

If you live in a dry/desert climate, exfoliate not only your face but also your entire body if possible (see Chapter 11/The Body), and always use a body moisturizer or oil. Dry hands also seem to be a frequent complaint with my Colorado clients. If you also have this problem, exfoliate your hands (especially the tops) and use a rich, moisturizing hand cream as often as possible. Remember to apply hand cream before you go to sleep. Don't leave your hands literally "high and dry" all night long.

Humid weather. Humidity, even on no-problem skin, can wreak havoc. Really humid weather can cause breakouts and irritations on the skin's surface even if there are usually no problems. The instructions for your skin in humid climates are about the same as for hot weather. Your skin is going to be excreting more sweat and oil and will tend to become more sticky and more oily than usual. So make sure to be diligent about your daily cleansing. If you're experiencing breakout, also use a clay mask two to three times per week if possible. Doing so will keep your skin from getting too congested, which can lead to breakouts. Drink lots of water and don't forget to exfoliate. If you have oily skin, you may want to find a moisturizing gel to replace your cream. Gels are lighter and won't feel as heavy as moisturizing creams. Keeping your skin clean, however, is your main priority.

Kick The Habit

Why do women wear foundation? Some wear it strictly out of habit. They automatically put it on without thinking. Others wear it because they are told they should. Many women wear foundation to even out their skin tone. Some women simply like to wear it.

At the cosmetic counter, the sales staff will tell you how good foundation is for your skin, how it contains sunscreen, protects you from the outside environment, and can help to even out your coloring. All of this is true. Many foundations do contain sunscreens, and using sunscreen is very important. Foundation does add another layer between you and the dirt, debris, and pollution in the air. Finally, foundation will even out your skin tone, and this is the benefit I want to discuss.

The meaning of the phrase *to even out skin tone* has eluded me for years. The skin all over your body has certain intrinsic characteristics to it—color, texture, moles, and freckles. Hardly anyone has totally "even" skin tone. Once in a while I come across someone who has perfect coloring, and inevitably even *she* has covered up perfection with foundation. A woman will make everything evened out on her face, while the rest of her body looks natural, having a flow to the tone and coloring of her skin. In other words, the skin on her body looks normal and unaffected. How many times have you seen a perfectly made-up face, then looked at that person's arms, shoulders, or neck only to see the skin's natural tone?

Foundation gives you a matte canvas on which to paint, a single-toned pallet to apply color to. Skin, however, is not usually this monochrome. It is full of imperfections and color differences, freckles, and pigmentation. I'm not talking about obvious, dark pigmentation spots or port-wine stains, for instance. I'm referring to women who have perfectly normal skin tone with naturally occurring pigmentation. Trying to cover up these small differences is, I believe, an attempt to cover up self-described flaws that I don't see as flaws at all. Wearing color (eyes, lips, cheeks) is fine. That's purely personal preference. Why can't we just stop there?

Foundation is actually *not* good for your skin. It acts as an occlusive covering over the skin. Its purpose is to remain on the surface, not to penetrate like a moisturizer. So it stays on top, just sitting there. As you now know, your skin doesn't breathe from the outside, so foundation doesn't keep your skin from breathing. It does, however, inhibit elimination. And your skin will absorb some of the foundation. After all, it's just sitting there all day long. Undoubtedly some of it will seep into your pores. And when this happens, the pores can enlarge. Foundation can cause congestion as well, especially if you have an oily skin type. If you have breakout and are using foundation, you are just fueling the very problem the foundation is attempting to cover up.

It's not as though you can wake up tomorrow and simply stop wearing it; foundation is a habit. Since you're used to seeing yourself look a certain way, I think weaning yourself off the look of foundation is the best way to change this particular habit. Start by adding water to your base makeup to thin it out. By the time you put foundation on this way, it's almost as though you have none on at all. So why wear it? Use this thinned-out foundation and gradually put less and less on until you're used to seeing your skin with hardly anything covering it. Eventually, just stop putting foundation on at all. Your eyes will have adjusted to what you're seeing in the mirror, and those around you will have adjusted to your new look as well.

All of the women I've encouraged to stop wearing foundation are ecstatic. They never thought they could go without, and now that they have, they love it! Their skin looks and feels better; they don't get foundation all over their clothes or worry if it needs touching up. They feel free and liberated.

Do you need to free yourself from this unnecessary step? Try to wean yourself off foundation and see how it goes. Worst case scenario—you go back to wearing it. But please know it serves no beneficial purpose to the skin. Or rather, any benefits you may derive from wearing foundation, like shielding you from the environment and adding an SPF to your skin, are totally outweighed by the detrimental effects, which are clogging, congestion, and enlarged pores. *Health* is the only foundation.

Standing Tall

Although posture is not a Forgotten Place like those listed in Chapter 12, good posture seems to be a forgotten practice I want to address. And although how good or bad your posture is doesn't directly affect your skin, it does affect your general and long-term health.

I find it so interesting how we carry ourselves. You can tell a lot about people by how they hold themselves up. Because we have to use our backs all of our lives, and because they tend to give us problems as we get older, I think it's important to take care of our backs now, so they will last for a lifetime. Exercise is always important, but posture and how we walk around all day long can affect the health of our backs as well. Taking a stand on proper posture is a good start toward taking good care of your back.

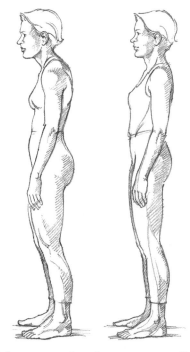

Start observing people, and you'll be amazed at how many of them are walking around hunched over or sunken in. I want to go over and gently pull them up to a straight and upright position. It's a bad habit, but I believe anyone can correct bad posture. (Obviously, I'm not talking about people who have chronic back trouble or spinal abnormalities.) Women are the worst when it comes to walking around with poor posture. I half-jokingly say, "If you want an instant breast lift, stand up straight."

When you're out, and you see someone with bad posture, use this as a signal to make sure you are standing tall. You can't go up to strangers and correct their posture, but you can use their example as a reminder to yourself to assume good posture. It's a minor correction that can help you look and feel better.

No Sweat

Anytime you sweat, especially from exercising, you don't want the sweat to dry on your skin. It contains acids and toxins that your body is trying to get rid of. When you are exercising outside, you're wearing sunscreen (I hope). So it's not only sweat that is going to clog your pores, but sweat mixed with sunscreen. It is imperative you don't let this mixture dry on your face. If you do, all that toxic junk sitting on your skin's surface will cause the potential for irritations, tiny bumps, and small whiteheads under your skin. These problems show up where the sweat drips—the sides of the neck, under the chin, and around the temples. If you are away from home but have access to water, great. Splash-rinse your face until you have removed all the sweaty residue off your skin. Then as soon as you get home, be sure and do your Basic 1-2-3 routine. Many of my active clients see a definite improvement in their skin after they use this splash-rinse method.

Sometimes you may be out exercising where you don't have access to water, yet you've got to get the sweat off your skin. If you cannot rinse your face, I am going to propose something to you that is *not* a great practice by any means, and certainly is not the optimum. However, the way I see it, it's the lesser of two evils.

After exercise that causes sweating (especially heavy sweating), and before the sweat starts to dry on your skin, use an individually wrapped moist towelette, facial cleansing cloth, or baby wipe tissue. Go over your entire face and neck, the back of your neck, and especially the sides of your neck. Keep in mind, this is only temporary until you get home and can properly clean your skin with good products. These towelettes usually have harsh ingredients in them (sometimes alcohol), but I believe it is better to get all the toxic, sweaty junk off your skin rather than let it dry on your face.

You will almost always have access to water, which is the best way to get the sweat off your face. So the moist towelette route would be the least-preferred way to go. I am not advocating their use all the time or even frequently. But if you have no other recourse (other than letting the sweat dry on your skin), use a towelette.

Keeping bottled water in your car is one way to ensure you will always be able to splash-rinse after exercising. Even if you're far from home (and your cleanser), at least you can get the sticky goo off your face and get home without causing the potential for breakouts. Keep in mind, you are rinsing everything, including sunscreen, off your face. Your skin, therefore, is totally unprotected. Running errands or otherwise being exposed to the sun is not recommended. Get home, clean your face, and apply sunscreen before going back outside.

The Next Best Thing

It's three o'clock in the afternoon, and you are in need of that cup of coffee or candy bar, whatever you reach for to get you through your afternoon slump. What you really need is a 15- or 20-minute nap. But that's absurd, right? You can't nap at the office or when the kids are on their way home from school. Yet that is exactly what your body needs. The very reason it is slowing down is because it's tired. Your body just needs a little refresher nap to get your batteries recharged, but you can't fit a nap in. (Older people and babies have the right idea—they take daily naps.)

My advice? Do the next best thing—whatever that looks like for you. Maybe you could close your office door and do a five-minute meditation to clear your thoughts and breathe. Or slip outside and find a private little spot to quiet your mind for five or ten minutes. Breathe in some clean air and let go of the day. Perhaps taking a walk can help you relax and release tension. If the kids are coming home at three every day, be home by 2:30 and take a 15-minute bath or sit and meditate for 15 minutes. If you don't have 15 minutes, then take five. Whatever the scenario, try to incorporate the next best thing into your day if you can't do what your body really wants to do, which is to rest and shut down for a while.

The same principle applies with exercise. Can't get your full workout in? Do the next best thing, which is perhaps only half your workout or one set of the exercises in your program. Maybe you can do a simple form of exercise instead of no exercise. The next best thing is always better than nothing at all.

With diet (your daily intake of food), again do the next best thing if you can't eat the best-quality food. If you want a snack and can't find fruit or other healthy foods to munch on, try a smoothie, crackers and cheese (easy to keep at the office), a glass of Emergen-C, or sparkling water with lemon. Anything other than cookies, candies, or other varieties of junk food will work. If you can't find a way to do the best thing in any given situation, do the next best thing.

All Stressed Out

When you're stressed, it's a time when your body needs three things: rest and relaxation; healthy, clean, and easy-to-digest foods; and water as the main source of fluids. However, when you're under stress you may tend to sleep less, eat poorly, and perhaps drink more alcohol (and/or coffee and sodas). So you may do the very things that will tax your body, making the stress even more significant.

This might be a good time to incorporate the next best thing into your day as much as possible. Taking supplements to help boost your weakened immune system would also be a good idea. Do anything you can in the course of your day that will help lessen the amount of stress you are feeling.

There are many people who do Chair Massage and will come to your office for a 15- or 30-minute "quicky" that can work wonders for relieving stress. Keeping good foods and clean water within close reach would also be helpful since stressful days usually mean you have less time to take for meals and snacks.

During periods of stress, the skin tends to suffer. Try to exfoliate regularly, and keep up with The Basics every day. Many of your routines may fall by the wayside when you are stressed, so try to keep up with at least a minimum of skin care instead of none at all. This would be a good time to get a facial. You can relax for an hour while someone takes good care of your skin.

There are many different, small things you can do to help your body get through the stresses of the day. Try to find at least one or two to help lessen the intensity of your day—every day. Including anti-stress activities can go a long way to helping you with short-term or even long-term stress in your life. Take care of your body now, so it can carry you through stressful times and lead you to the light at the end of the tunnel.

Fragrances of Old

Perfumeries started out using pure essential oils and floral waters as fragrances way back when. Then with the arrival of science, synthetic fragrances were born. Most perfumes today are made up predominantly or entirely of synthetics. Synthetics are usually cheaper ingredients and can be an affront to your senses. When pure essences are used, you are getting a pleasant scent and sensation although you are going to pay premium prices for this all-natural interlude.

With strong, synthetic fragrances, your olfactory (smell) glands go into overdrive, and many times a headache will follow. Many people get headaches simply from walking through the department store cosmetic and fragrance areas, especially when the salespeople are so eagerly spraying perfumes at you left and right.

When fragrance is used as an ingredient in skin care products, you may get headaches from this as well. You may experience topical intolerances such as red, rashy skin, or even breakout. This can be due to an allergic response or intolerance to a particular fragrance.

Because how a product smells greatly influences your desire to purchase it, companies will put their trademark fragrance in most or all of their skin care products, hoping to entice you to buy them. If you are not sensitive to fragrance, these products will probably not cause you problems. But if you are sensitive, watch out. It won't take long for your skin to give you a clear and unmistakable signal that it does not like a product you're using.

Pay attention to any warning signs (redness, itching, irritation, rashes, breakout) when using a new skin care product. If it contains fragrance, you may have to opt for a more natural product, one that utilizes natural fragrances, such as essential oils. (See Chapter 8/ Essential Oils.) These natural essences give products wonderful aromas without the irritations caused by synthetic fragrances.

Pillow Talk

Lavender is known as a soothing and calming essential oil. It has a pleasant aroma, one almost everyone is familiar with. If you are having trouble sleeping, one helpful remedy would be to put a few drops of essential oil of lavender on your pillow (or on a handkerchief), and let the relaxing melody of this essence soothe you to sleep. It makes a nice addition to your travel bag since traveling often means a poor night's sleep.

Lavender is also very soothing to burns. For instance, if you have burned yourself on a hot stove or an iron, lavender will quickly take out the burning sensation. My number one recommendation for sunburns is aloe vera gel (see Chapter 10), but for any other kind of burn lavender works wonders.

Stop Bugging Me

Bug bites? Have I got the answer for you! Essential oil of peppermint is the fastest (and most aromatic) way to stop the itching of a bug bite. Just put a drop on any mosquito, chigger, or flea bite and within a few seconds, the itching will stop. I've even put it on nasty fire ant bites (the kind that hurt) with great results. Although peppermint oil is best for relieving the sting and itch of bug bites, lavender can also do a good job.

Another wonderful use for peppermint oil: put a drop in your mouth and wait to be refreshed. It's better than any breath mint or mouthwash you can imagine. I like to apply it to a Q-tip, and then swab the inside of my mouth. A little peppermint oil goes a long way.

A few words of caution: *never* get peppermint oil in or around your eyes. It will burn like nothing you've ever known before! As with all essential oils, never get them near your eyes, but especially peppermint oil. This is one reason I like to use a Q-tip when applying this oil. Then I won't accidentally get the peppermint on my fingers and inadvertently rub my eyes at some point afterwards.

Hangover Helpers

Alcohol has a definite effect on your skin. If you're going to drink, incorporating the following steps will not only help replace lost nutrients and water in your alcohol-depleted skin, these suggestions will also help curb some of the "morning after" problems you may encounter. It is preferable to attend to this the night you do the drinking instead of waiting for the morning after. But in case you weren't able to get to your cure the night before, take these steps in the morning—first thing after waking if possible. Nothing will completely eliminate the ill effects alcohol can have on your skin (and your entire body), but hopefully these will help lessen the negative effects and make the next day a productive one.

Water. Try to drink two glasses of water for every glass of alcohol you drink. Although this method is optimum, it may be an impossible request. At least try to get one glass of water for each alcoholic drink. Alcohol is a diuretic and causes dehydration throughout your entire system. Add to that the toxic nature of alcohol, and your body is in serious need of fluids. And the body's fluid of choice? Plain, clean water. Even if you're just having a glass of wine with dinner, drink a few extra glasses of water. It will help to replace what is being taken out of your body (and your skin) from alcohol consumption.

Evening primrose oil. As mentioned in Chapter 14, taking a few evening primrose capsules (six to ten) before bed can go a long way to curbing a hangover.

Emergen-C. There are many uses for Emergen-C (see Chapter 14), but I highly recommend taking it before bed and upon arising after a night of drinking. Even if you didn't drink heavily, Emergen-C contains vitamins, minerals, and electrolytes that are lost through the consumption of alcohol, no matter how little. If you're hungover, the fizzy nature of Emergen-C can help to quench the inevitable thirst that hits you in the middle of the night and the next morning. Hopefully you drank enough water during your night out to help keep dehydration at bay, but Emergen-C will help to replace lost elements and hopefully help to get you back on your feet again.

Constipation

We freely and easily talk about what we're putting into our bodies, but rarely if ever do we discuss elimination. However you want to portray the event, proper elimination is essential to a healthy body and, therefore, healthy skin. All of your eliminating organs need to be functioning optimally for the toxins in your body to be dealt with and removed. If your colon is sluggish, sooner or later there will be trouble. Have you ever forgotten to take out your kitchen garbage? You can smell the gases and toxins building up inside the plastic. Your colon goes through a similar process when you are constipated. Like the garbage, food that is stuck in your colon will ferment and cause noxious gases to form. These gases keep building up until the waste is removed. In the meantime, the toxins can be reabsorbed into your system and released through your skin (the largest organ of elimination).

So what's the solution? There are several answers to this question. The first thing I recommend is to read about colon health, so you will have a better understanding of this barely talked about but vital process. I have listed several helpful books at the end of this chapter.

Water. Water. Water. One reason your bowels aren't moving might be because your large intestine has become dehydrated. Your body requires adequate amounts of water in order to pass waste through the length of your intestines. The best way to get water into your system is to *drink water*. Anytime I have clients who complain of constipation, I instruct them to start drinking more water. Water is essential in helping to relieve constipation. (See Chapter 14/Water.)

Chlorophyll is another key ingredient when it comes to colon health. If a client comes to me with a lot of blemishes, I inquire about the possibility of constipation. The colon contains a lot of toxins that can get reabsorbed into the bloodstream and come out of your skin as breakout. Chlorophyll helps to loosen hardened matter off the colon wall and gets debris moving through the intestines. Taking chlorophyll is an excellent way to get things cleared out of your colon, and therefore, your skin. (See Chapter 14/Chlorophyll.)

Eating high-quality foods for colon health goes without saying (I hope). Poor-quality foods (fast-foods, for instance) and low water-content foods (basically anything that isn't a fruit or vegetable) take a lot of water to digest. Fruits and vegetables not only contain a lot of water but are also good sources of vitamins and minerals.

Exercise is another key to healthy bowel movements. Peristalsis (the muscular contractions that occur in your large intestine to move waste toward its final destination) is stimulated with exercise. Aside from toning your legs and other muscles, exercise (even simply walking) helps to tone your inner organs as well, which includes your colon. Walking is one of the best and easiest ways to tone your body and help alleviate constipation. If you are constipated, start walking, drinking more water, taking chlorophyll, and eating high water-content foods. See if this helps to lessen your troubles.

Suggested Reading

The Art of Doing Nothing by Veronique Vienne (New York: Clarkson Potter/Publishers, 1998). This wonderful little book (complete with beautiful photography) has great tips on how to make time for yourself.

Healing Within: The Complete Guide To Colon Health by Stanley Weinberger (Larkspur, CA: Healing Within Products, 1996). A good book to help you understand the correlation between colon health and feeling vibrant.

The Natural Guide To Colon Health by Louise Tenney, M.H., with Deanne Tenney (Pleasant Grove, UT: Woodland Publishing, 1997). Another informative book on how to keep your colon healthy.

Posture Makes Perfect by Dr. Victor Barker (New York: Japan Publications, Inc., 1993). This is the quintessential book about posture. It is fully illustrated and fascinating.

16

Common Myths Dispelled

There are many falsehoods floating around in the skin care world. Quick fixes don't work, and neither do miracle regimens. And remember, if something sounds too good to be true, it probably is. With all the myths circulating about caring for the skin, it's bound to get confusing. What should you believe? My best advice to you is this: use your common sense. Claims and promises seduce you into buying products; they don't necessarily bring you the promised results. Start now (or continue) to affect your skin in a healthy way by following The Basics and The Extras along with other suggestions in this book.

Before and after pictures. I never consider these types of photographs when determining the effectiveness of a treatment or product and I highly recommend you don't either. The variables that are possible with before and after pictures are numerous. Lighting, camera angles, clothing color, hairstyle, and even facial expressions can all make the image look better or worse depending on what is needed. I like to turn the photos upside down to lose (or gain) perspective. Remember, these are advertisements meant to sell you something. Please don't use these pictures as a basis for believing anything.

Chocolate makes your skin break out. It's not the cocoa in chocolate that makes your skin break out. But when you eat chocolate, it is inevitably made with sugar (like a candy bar), and it is the *sugar* that is most likely causing the breakout. So this myth is partially true, depending on how you are defining chocolate. (See Chapter 13/Sugar.)

European facials. Europe is known for its product lines. Skin care really began in Europe, as did the utilization of spas, going to the baths, hydrotherapy, etc. But to characterize something as being *European* should not be an automatic cinch for a service or person being of high quality. To me, the phrase *European facial* would indicate a facial given in Europe. I suppose it could be a facial given by a European aesthetician, or perhaps the product that is being used is from Europe. But I really think it's a meaningless term used to elevate the quality of a facial treatment.

Many times the word *European* is used to connote some special, sophisticated training. Training is obviously very important, but where the education takes place doesn't necessarily mean it was or was not good training. Quality depends on many factors. It is the talent of the individual along with education and training that creates a good aesthetician.

So when a salon says it offers a European facial, ask "What exactly does that mean?" For example, I am an American, trained in America, using French products. Am I giving a European facial?

Facial exercises help reduce wrinkles and/or firm the skin. Wrinkles are lines of expression. They are formed by the constant animation of your face. Most of these facial exercise regimens encourage you to make faces that, I hate to tell you, are just increasing the depth and premature appearance of lines on your face. Don't rush your wrinkles!

Facials make your skin break out. You'll sometimes hear how getting a facial helps bring the impurities in your skin to the surface. Therefore if you experience breakout after a facial, it's actually a good thing. Well, I disagree. True, once in a while getting a facial may speed up the elimination of one or two small places on your face. But facials really should clear up your skin, not cause breakout. Perhaps you are having a reaction to the products used. Perhaps the aesthetician extracted too many places, which caused irritation and inflammation. But if you had an effective facial treatment, it is my belief that your skin should reflect this by looking clean, clear, and free from new breakout. Anything more than a small place or two every once in a while after a facial is indicative of a problem with the facial or the products, not with your skin.

Facial tissue (Kleenex) **is bad for your skin.** Because tissues are made from wood pulp, it is said they can scratch your skin. Personally, I think this is ridiculous. You may be using an abrasive scrub on your face, yet you are told to worry about using facial tissue! So if you choose to use tissues, don't think you are harming your skin. Obviously, softer tissues will feel better than the cheaper, coarser types. Either way, feel free to use tissue if you need to. I am not, however, a fan of tissuing things off your face. Instead, you want to rinse products off by using your hands to ensure everything has been removed.

Foundation is good for the skin. As you've read in the previous chapter, foundation is not the most beneficial product to use on your skin. It can clog your pores, inhibit elimination, and cover up your natural skin tone.

It's expensive, so it must be good. True, most good products cost more than the average grocery or department store brand, but not always. Just because something is expensive doesn't automatically mean it is a quality product. You may just be paying for the brand name, the attractive packaging, or expensive advertising. Don't be fooled by the price tag. The proof will always be in the results you receive.

My skin is dry. Many times dry skin is simply dehydrated skin. True-dry skin is not as common as you might think. This distinction becomes important when shopping for products. Read over Chapter 4 on skin types to get detailed information to help you understand these two different types of skin.

Night creams need to be heavy. Night creams don't have to be heavy. They commonly are, which can lead to breakout or just a feeling of greasiness. Ingredients in night treatments are usually more regenerative and repairing, but they need not be heavy. There is a long-standing image of our grandmothers going to bed with a heavy layer of greasy cream on their faces. Somehow manufacturers have not completely gotten away from this image and still make night creams that are heavy and greasy. Just know your night cream is more of a treatment cream and should be designed to tackle problems specific to your skin type (sensitive, couperose, dry, oily, problem, etc.). This does not have to affect the thickness of the cream, however.

Oily skin wrinkles less. Lines and wrinkles are formed from a breakdown in collagen fibers over a long period of expressing, sun exposure, and just plain time. Oily skin does keep a lipid or oily film over the face, which does keep it moisturized and supple. The sebaceous or oil glands, however, have nothing to do with collagen fibers.

Oily skin tends to be thick skin; thick skin ages differently. It tends to form one or two deep wrinkles, whereas thin skin usually has many very fine lines. Think of a piece of heavy wool versus a thin piece of silk. When folded, the wool will only crease in one or two places, but the creases will be deep. The silk may form many creases, but they will be superficial.

The oil content of your skin has very little to do with the aging process. Accumulated sun exposure, genetics, and how expressive you are determine how your lines will form.

Pores shrink. The plain truth is this: pores don't shrink. There is no cream, ointment, or skin care regimen that can change this fact. Pores are not little openings that can expand and contract like muscles. They do expand or stretch, but pores are not so elastic that they can contract to their former, smaller state.

Pores will naturally enlarge as you get older due to the downward pull of gravity (especially in the cheek area). Because oily skin is usually congested, this type of skin will be more prone to enlarged pores. Debris nestled in the pores over a period of time will expand the opening to support the enlarging plug or blackhead. Your Extras routine, done on a regular basis, will help keep dead skin and oil from clogging your pores and lessen the chance of enlargement.

Preventing wrinkles. You may hear and see ads about how cream "X" prevents wrinkles. Well, no cream or product you can buy will truly prevent what nature has in store for you. Is there anything you can do to lessen their appearance? Yes. (1) Stay away from direct sunlight. This is one surefire way to actually prevent wrinkles. (2) Get into good skin care habits early. Any care you give your skin will be reciprocated in kind by healthy tissue and cells. (3) Don't drink alcohol or smoke. (4) Pick parents with good genes for skin. First it is genetics, then sun exposure, and finally the care you take of your skin that are the keys to preventing or causing wrinkles.

Products can firm your skin. It is physiologically impossible to firm tissue. Short of stretching the skin through plastic surgery, the skin's elasticity cannot be restored once it has become flaccid. Like a rubber band, once the tissue has lost that bounce-back ability, firm skin is a thing of the past.

Skin breathes. As I discussed at the beginning of Chapter 1, your skin doesn't have little noses on the outside breathing in oxygen. Your skin is nourished by the oxygen carried in the blood. Products, therefore, don't stop your skin from breathing.

Soap is a good cleanser. Soap, because of its alkaline nature, strips your skin of all oil and water and sets up an imbalanced environment usually leading to dehydration and possibly congestion. (See Chapter 1/Cleansing: What to use.)

Sun clears up acne. I've seen books that were published in the late '70s through the early '80s that actually have chapters on "safe suntanning." Other chapters suggest lying out in the sun to help clear acne. Well, no amount of sun is really good for your skin. And certainly sun doesn't control acne. What sun exposure can do is put some skin problems in a dormant state, only to have these trouble spots reactivate at a later date. Sun will dry out the outer skin, which has a temporary effect of drying, as well as a psychological effect of clearing. But as far as being a treatment for problem skin, sun exposure won't do the trick. Heat actually *activates* your oil glands. So lying out in the sun to clear up acne is probably, in the long run, going to increase any existing problems.

Tanned skin is healthy skin. This is one of the biggest myths around. It's true that when you get a tan, you may feel healthier. And I must admit, you tend to look healthier with a little bit of color. However, the truth is (as you have read in Chapter 10) that the color change in your skin called a tan is actually the body's response to danger—danger from the harmful rays of the sun. If having a tan is important to you, just remember you are incurring sun-time that, as you get older, will show up as sun damage. Sun damage could be anything from loose, sagging skin; permanent redness (couperose); or, worst case scenario, skin cancer. The truth is, suntanned skin is sun-damaged skin.

Toners are the second step in cleansing. Toners have nothing to do with cleansing your skin. They are used to superficially hydrate the outer skin, reacidify the epidermis, and prepare the skin for moisturizer. (For more details see Chapter 1/Toning: Why use a toner?)

Use a separate cream for your neck. Neck or throat creams are another ploy to get you to buy more products. Although the skin on your neck varies from the skin on your face, I recommend treating it basically the same. Include your neck in everything you do, The Basics 1-2-3 plus exfoliation and sunscreen. It is usually unnecessary to purchase a separate cream for this area.

17

Ageless Beauty

Although each part of this book is valuable, this last chapter is in many ways the most important. Discussing care of your skin from the outside is pretty straightforward. When you adopt a particular suggestion, there will be a probable outcome. But skin care in regard to aging is not purely topical. I cannot separate the importance of taking care of your skin from the inside (both inside your body *and* your mind) and topical care. Talking about healing from deep within becomes a bit complex, and that is what this chapter is all about.

I truly believe aging is not the terrible thing it is represented to be in the consciousness of this country. Aging is inevitable, and it is the most natural process in life—one to be heralded, not condemned. A pervasive perception in our society today is that there is something inherently wrong with getting older. Yes, it can be disheartening to see the lines start to form or get deeper. Slowing down, losing your 20/20 vision, and waking up to stiff joints are not what you would choose for yourself. Although degenerating is the part of the process that is perhaps the hardest to take, what about what you gain with age?

The big question is "What is wrong with aging?" If you spend your whole life fighting the aging process, are you really living? What are you comparing old to? How will *you* grow old? Do you know older people who seem young? People who haven't caved in to some society-driven illusion of how "old is bad." The adage about wine getting better with time—isn't this true for people as well?

Aging with grace is what I'm striving for in my own life, and it is what I discuss with my clients. You can struggle with what is happening and put up a big fight, but the bottom line is the aging of your body will occur anyway. There are no miracles to be found in a jar of cream, nor is there a Fountain of Youth at the doctor's office. You are your own living miracle, and how your body functions is the daily affirmation, the absolute proof. The Fountain of Youth is inside you.

What do you see when you look in the mirror? I'd like to think you see a beautiful soul living each day to the fullest, doing the best you can in any given situation. In other words, you see your humanness. I have a feeling, however, some of you see something completely different. Maybe you see someone you wish you weren't. Perhaps you are comparing yourself to your skinny neighbor or your friends with flawless skin. When you look in the mirror, do you see your true self or only someone in comparison to someone else?

It's a simple matter of "compare and despair." If you are constantly comparing yourself to other people (who, by the way, are comparing themselves to *their* ideal), you will never be happy or satisfied with the way you look. How could you possibly compare? They are "ideal," "perfect," "without flaws." It's as though there is something wrong with feeling OK about the way you look!

How you see yourself is relative. It's relative to how you feel. It's relative to what you want to look like in comparison to what you do look like. When have you ever looked in the mirror on a day you felt horrible and said, "I look great today!"? Probably never! But conversely, haven't you looked in the mirror on a day when everything was going your way and said, "Hey, I look pretty good!"? Well, these days can occur back to back, one after the other. One day you're up; the next you're down. And so too is how you see yourself. But physically, your body (your face) doesn't change overnight. Rarely do significant changes occur, even over a short period of time. It's all in your attitude and how you feel that gets projected onto the image you see in the mirror.

The funny thing about worrying over how we look is that everyone else (almost everyone) has similar feelings about themselves. A client came to me years ago, distraught about a "huge" pimple on her face. (*Huge* to her was not *huge* to me.) She was going to a black tie affair and was so worried about what everyone would think about her blemish. As I worked on her skin, I reminded her that more than likely everyone would be worried about themselves, totally missing her "big zit." Perhaps they might have spilled something on their clothes on the way to the party or couldn't get their hair to do the right thing. It would be doubtful that other people would be focusing on something wrong with my client. More than likely, they would be worried about something in their own appearances.

Call me crazy, but in my perfect world people aren't worried about what they look like so much as who they are. How you present yourself to the world is measured (in my mind) by your character. The question I ask myself is, "Am I a good person?" not "Am I good-looking?"

I think if we lived in a world without mirrors we would think differently about who we are. We wouldn't be able to look in the mirror and pick ourselves apart, condemning what nature or our parents gave us. We would accept our looks because we wouldn't be able to compare them to anyone else's. And certainly there would be no comparisons to supermodels gracing the pages of fashion magazines and TV commercials.

What you get out of life tends to be measured by what you put into it. (In physics it's known as the law of cause and effect.) Regarding aging, genetics start things off. But if you are blessed with good genes and consistently don't take care of your body, history will eventually tell the real story by your state of health. This is true for your skin as well. If you do all the right things, you will most likely receive the payoff. The tough realization is youth will not come from a single bottle, a magic potion, and in my opinion not even through cosmetic surgery.

What causes you to age is not just the natural degeneration of your cells, but your inner thoughts as well. Choosing how you age, acknowledging your inner beauty, accepting the process, and deciding to age with grace are internal factors that can have a positive impact on how you feel about aging (on the inside), which affects how you will age (on the outside).

Choosing how you age. When you look in the mirror, you make a choice (consciously or unconsciously) to either like and accept what you see or not to like it. If you choose not to accept something, lines and wrinkles for instance, you've got a problem. And a problem begs for a solution. Some of the possible solutions are discussed in Chapter 9. However, you have the answers inside of you. In order to resolve this conflict, it will require discipline and a paradigm shift. If you change the way you see yourself, you can change how you age. To some, this may seem like a simplistic approach. But committing to changing your attitude—your inner dialogue—can profoundly affect every aspect of your personal and individual aging process.

What you spend your time thinking about is what you will eventually create (attract) in your life. Why not choose thoughts that are healing and kind versus negative and hurtful? It is a *choice*. How you see the world and how the world sees you (through your most constant thoughts) is up to you. If you believe you look bad, ugly, or aged, that will be your experience when you're out in the world. If you choose to see your beauty, the world will reflect this thought back to you.

If throughout our lives all we ever heard was how great it was to be old, how cool wrinkles were, and how we'd gain wisdom and stability with age, we'd be totally into growing older. Reverse all that, and it's the way we think about aging today. Like many things in life, your attitude comes down to choice. Will you choose to deny or abhor aging? Or will you choose to acknowledge all the good that comes with those wrinkles? What if wrinkles *were* cool? That attitude shift can change your life. It is within your power to create new thoughts to promote your well-being. I believe this with all my heart.

Acknowledging your inner beauty. Have you ever met someone who wasn't physically beautiful but had an inner beauty so radiant and so strong, it made this person beautiful in all ways? It really is your *inner* beauty that makes you attractive, beautiful, and radiant. Without the acknowledgment of your inner beauty, you are just an empty shell. Perhaps a physically attractive shell, but a hollow and vacant shell nonetheless. Being able to recognize your inner self (your beauty from within) isn't easy. It takes work. But if you commit to discovering and developing this part of yourself, the rewards are immeasurable.

It's a never-ending process. You won't wake up one day and forevermore not need to work on keeping a positive attitude. You won't suddenly look in the mirror and think you're utter perfection. It's a constant and unending effort to not give in to your negative, self-condemning thoughts and to raise yourself up to a different level. It takes strength to keep yourself on track. And just like exercising your muscles to keep them strong, you have to exercise your desire to see your inner beauty. You have to exercise your belief in that timeless, ageless aspect of yourself. Without this persistent pursuit, your will and determination will atrophy and wither away, just like your muscles do without exercise.

Acceptance. Our first inclination is to resist aging. Then, for some, comes the reluctant acceptance of the changes aging brings. For others, it's time for "The Big Fight," electing to change the outside through surgery or other invasive procedures. At some point the decision of how to deal with what we've got (or lost) will come about for everyone. I propose, whether you change the outside or not, to commit to changing your inside first. Changing your attitude toward yourself, plus truly accepting the aging process. This isn't about giving up, it's about acknowledging the reality of life and finding beauty and positive things therein. This is a strange concept in comparison to the predominant trend of cutting and sewing and pasting ourselves back to being young. I gladly go against the grain.

When you look at photos of yourself from when you were younger, is that the look you are trying to bring back into your life? When I see pictures of myself in my 20s, I look like a baby—no wrinkles and flawless skin. But who was I? A naive young woman struggling on a daily basis to find her place in the world. Now years later, I no longer battle the angst of youth I used to. What a pleasure! And with this inner stability I have gained comes exterior signs of maturity as well—wrinkles, less elastic skin, pockets of fat that just won't go away. One goes hand in hand with the other—wisdom and experience along with various signs of aging.

Acceptance of aging (for me) means embracing the process instead of running from it. I don't really like to see the lines etching themselves into my face, but I have chosen to accept their presence and acknowledge their beauty. This is a conscious decision of acceptance; one I continually make. I choose to see these etchings as markers of my growth in life. In other words, they don't take anything away from me; these lines add to who I am. I want to go through life finding positive ways to see the changes that are taking place, rather than pursuing the alternatives. It really is a creative process—trying to find new and positive ways to look at the aging process as it unfolds.

Aging with grace. Acknowledging your inner beauty and accepting the natural aging process is what aging with grace is all about. It is not about bowing down to the outside world, but drawing strength from within. Whether or not you have had or are planning cosmetic surgery, it is never too late to start working on the inside; the inner, all-knowing voice that says you are OK just exactly the way you are. Slow, methodical, internal changes can actually result in long-term benefits—given a chance.

The bottom line is you will do exactly what you want to do. This may mean having surgery to get back something you feel you've lost (or never had in the first place). It may mean choosing to find the positive aspects of aging naturally. Whichever path you choose in your life, I wish you well. Serenity may come from cosmetic changes; however, I believe true peace comes from doing inner work. It takes longer and seems to be much more difficult than the quick-fix alternatives, but the benefits are everlasting. The results from changing the inside of who you are will in turn change how the world sees you. It's a beautiful thing.

May health, clear skin, and a feeling of inner peace be yours—for a lifetime.

Are You Considering Cosmetic Surgery? by Arthur W. Perry, M.D., and Robin K. Levinson. New York: Avon Books, 1997.

Aromatherapy: The Complete Guide to Plant & Flower Essences for Health & Beauty by Daniele Ryman. New York: Bantam Books, 1993.

The Beauty Bible by Paula Begoun. Seattle, Washington: Beginning Press, 1997.

The Complete Idiot's Guide to Beautiful Skin by Marsha Gordon, M.D., and Alice E. Fugate. New York: Alpha Books, 1998.

Evening Primrose Oil by Judy Graham. Rochester, Vermont: Thorson's Publishing Group, 1990.

Get The Sugar Out: 501 Simple Ways to Cut the Sugar Out of Any Diet by Louise Gittleman, M.S., C.N.S. New York: Three Rivers Press, 1996.

Healthy Skin, The Facts by Rona M. Mackie. Oxford: Oxford University Press, 1992.

The How To Herb Book by Velma J. Keith and Monteen Gordon. Pleasant Grove, UT: Mayfield Publications, 1994.

Merck Manual of Medical Information, Home Edition. New Jersey: Merck Research Laboratories, 1997.

Natural Health, Natural Medicine: A Comprehensive Manual for Wellness and Self-Care by Andrew Weil, M.D. New York: Houghton Mifflin Company, 1998.

The New Beacon Book of Quotations by Women by Rosalie Maggio. Boston: Beacon Press, 1996.

Taber's Cyclopedic Medical Dictionary. Philadelphia: F.A. Davis Company, 1997.

Take Care of Your Skin by Elaine Brumberg. New York: Harper Row, 1989.

A Woman Doctor's Guide to Skin Care by Wilma F. Bergfeld, M.D., F.A.C.P., with Shelagh Ryan Masline. New York: Hyperion, 1995.

Your Skin by Joseph P. Bark, M.D. New Jersey: Prentice Hall, 1995.

The Youth Corridor by Gerald Imber, M.D. New York: William Morrow and Company, Inc., 1997.

Carolyn Ash has been helping people with their skin for over 15 years. Her clientele ranges from celebrities to men and women in the workplace as well as teenagers with problem skin. Carolyn has developed a unique philosophy on caring for the skin that has worked for people of all ages. She currently operates Carolyn Ash Skin Care in Dallas, Texas. Carolyn's dedication to her profession is obvious in the loyalty exhibited by her clients.

Keep an eye out for future publications by Carolyn Ash, including a follow-up to *Timeless Skin*, entitled *Skin Care Q & A*. To contact Carolyn and to ask questions that may be included in her upcoming book, write to her at:

Carolyn Ash
c/o Splash Publishing
P.O. Box 720177
Dallas Texas 75372

or visit her website:
www.timelessskin.com